MW01233701

Peanut Butter Cookbook

125+ Irresistible Recipes to Make Every Brekfast Unforgettable

Robert Snearl

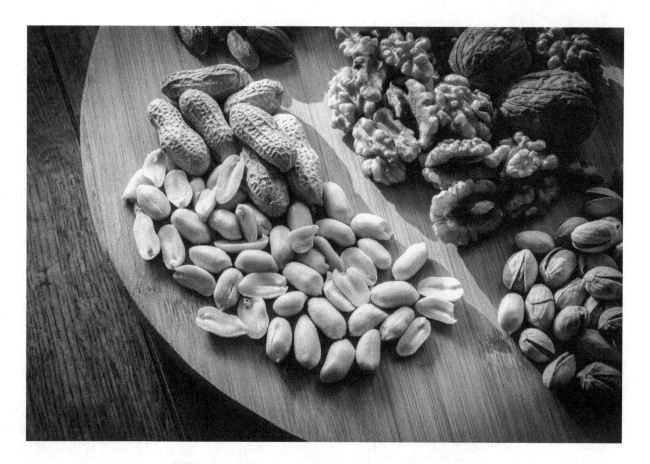

SPECIAL DISCLAIMER

All the information's included in this book are given for instructive, informational and entertainment purposes, the author can claim to share very good quality recipes but is not headed for the perfect data and uses of the mentioned recipes, in fact the information's are not intent to provide dietary advice without a medical consultancy.

The author does not hold any responsibility for errors, omissions or contrary interpretation of the content in this book.

It is recommended to consult a medical practitioner before to approach any kind of diet, especially if you have a particular health situation, the author isn't headed for the responsibility of these situations and everything is under the responsibility of the reader, the author strongly recommend to preserve the health taking all precautions to ensure ingredients are fully cooked.

All the trademarks and brands used in this book are only mentioned to clarify the sources of the information's and to describe better a topic and all the trademarks and brands mentioned own their copyrights and they are not related in any way to this document and to the author.

This document is written to clarify all the information's of publishing purposes and cover any possible issue.

This document is under copyright and it is not possible to reproduce any part of this content in every kind of digital or printable document. All rights reserved.

© Copyright 2021 Robert Snearl. All rights reserved.

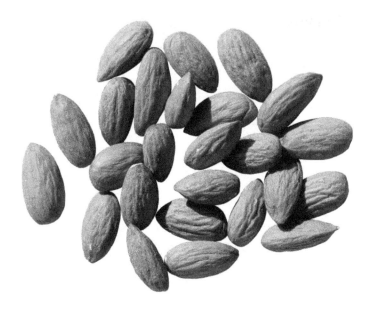

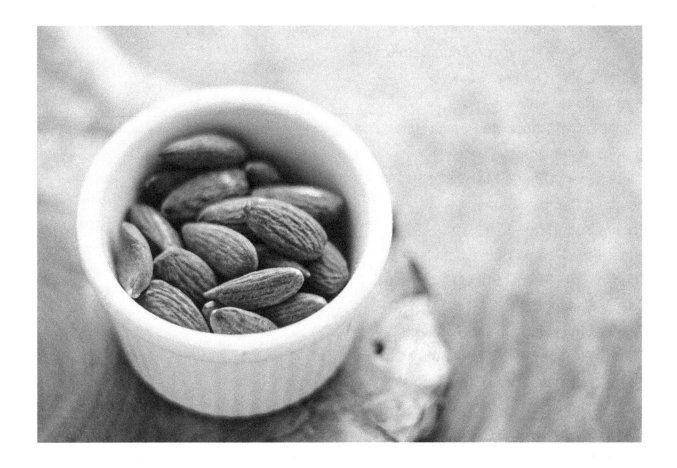

Table Of Contents

Table Of Contents

Table Of Contents

Table Of Contents

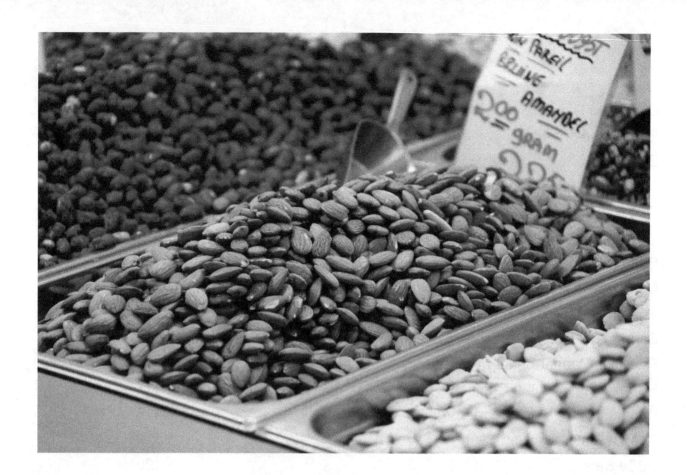

Chewy Chocolate Peanut Butter Chip Cookies

Ingredients

1 1/2 cups butter, melted
2 cups white sugar
2 eggs
1 teaspoon vanilla extract
2 cups all-purpose flour
3/4 cup unsweetened cocoa powder
1 teaspoon baking soda
1/2 teaspoon salt
2 cups peanut butter chips

Directions

Preheat oven to 350 degrees F (175 degrees C).

In a large bowl, mix together butter and sugar. Beat in eggs and vanilla. Combine flour, cocoa, baking soda, and salt; gradually stir into the butter mixture. Mix in peanut butter chips. Drop by rounded teaspoons onto ungreased cookie sheets.

Bake 8 to 10 minutes in preheated oven. Cool for 1 minute before placing on wire racks to cool completely.

Peanut Butter Maple Cookies

Ingredients

1 cup butter or margarine, softened
1/2 cup peanut butter*
1 cup sugar
1 cup packed brown sugar
2 eggs
1 tablespoon maple syrup
2 teaspoons vanilla extract
2 cups all-purpose flour
3/4 cup quick-cooking oats
1 1/2 teaspoons baking powder
1 teaspoon baking soda
1 teaspoon salt
1 (10 ounce) package peanut butter chips

Directions

In a mixing bowl, cream the butter, peanut butter and sugars. Add the eggs, one at a time, beating well after each addition. Beat in syrup and vanilla. Combine the flour, oats, baking powder, baking soda and salt; add to the creamed mixture and mix well. Stir in peanut butter chips.

Drop by heaping tablespoonfuls 2 in. apart onto ungreased baking sheets. Bake at 325 degrees F for 15-18 minutes or until golden brown. Cool for 1 minute before removing to wire racks.

Microwave Peanut Butter S'Mores

Ingredients

Graham crackers
JIF® Creamy Peanut Butter
Milk chocolate candy bars
Large marshmallows

Directions

Spread graham cracker square with peanut butter.

Top with a square of chocolate and a marshmallow.

Microwave on HIGH (100% power) 5 to 10 seconds or until marshmallow puffs.

Top with another cracker square. Serve immediately.

Banana Tortilla Snacks

Ingredients

1 (6 inch) flour tortilla
2 tablespoons peanut butter
1 tablespoon honey
1 banana
2 tablespoons raisins

Directions

Lay tortilla flat. Spread peanut butter and honey on tortilla. Place banana in the middle and sprinkle in the raisins. Wrap, and serve.

Peanut Butter Pinwheels

Ingredients

1/2 cup shortening
1/2 cup creamy peanut butter
1 cup sugar
1 egg
2 tablespoons milk
1 1/4 cups all-purpose flour
1/2 teaspoon baking soda
1/2 teaspoon salt
1 cup semisweet chocolate chips

Directions

In a mixing bowl, cream shortening, peanut butter and sugar. Beat in egg and milk. Combine the flour, baking soda and salt; gradually add to creamed mixture. Roll out between waxed paper into a 12-in. x 10-in. rectangle. Melt chocolate chips; cool slightly. Spread over dough to within 1/2 in. of edges. Roll up tightly, jelly-roll style, starting with a long side; wrap in plastic wrap. Refrigerate for 20-30 minutes or until easy to handle.

Unwrap dough and cut into 1/2-in. slices. Place 1 in. apart on greased baking sheets. Bake at 375 degrees F for 10-12 minutes or until edges are lightly browned. Remove to wire racks to cool.

Peanut Crumb Apple Pie

Ingredients

1 cup all-purpose flour
1/2 cup SMUCKER'S® Creamy Natural Peanut Butter
1/2 cup firmly packed light brown sugar
1/4 cup butter or margarine, softened
1/4 teaspoon salt
1 (30 ounce) can apple pie filling
1 (9 inch) unbaked pie shell

Directions

Blend flour, peanut butter, brown sugar, butter and salt until mixture is crumbly. Spoon apple pie filling into unbaked crust; sprinkle peanut butter mixture over pie filling.

Bake at 400 degrees F for 30 to 35 minutes or until filling is hot and pastry is browned.

Out-on-the-Range Cookies

Ingredients

3/4 cup shortening
1 1/4 cups packed brown sugar
1 cup sugar
2 eggs
1 cup peanut butter
1 teaspoon vanilla extract
1 3/4 cups all-purpose flour
1 cup quick-cooking oats
2 teaspoons baking soda
1/2 teaspoon salt
1 cup semisweet chocolate chips

Directions

In a mixing bowl, cream shortening and sugars. Add eggs, one at a time, beating well after each addition. Beat in peanut butter and vanilla. Combine the flour, oats, baking soda and salt; gradually add to the creamed mixture. Stir in chips.

Drop by rounded tablespoonfuls 2 in. apart onto greased baking sheets. Bake at 325 degrees F for 12-14 minutes or until golden brown. Remove to wire racks to cool.

Peanut Butter Puddingwiches

Ingredients

1 1/2 cups peanut butter, divided
3 cups cold milk, divided
1 (3.9 ounce) package instant chocolate pudding mix
2 cups whipped topping, divided
1 (3.4 ounce) package instant vanilla pudding mix
32 whole graham crackers

Directions

Line two 13-in. x 9-in. x 2-in. pans with foil; set aside. In a mixing bowl, combine 3/4 cup peanut butter and 1-1/2 cups milk until smooth. Slowly beat in chocolate pudding mix until blended; fold in 1 cup whipped topping. Pour into one prepared pan; freeze until firm. Repeat with vanilla pudding and remaining peanut butter, milk and whipped topping. Pour into second pan; freeze until firm.

Break or cut graham crackers into squares. Cut frozen pudding mixture into 32 squares, about 2-1/2 in. x 2-1/4 in.; place each square between two crackers. Wrap in plastic wrap. Freeze overnight.

Classic Peanut Butter Cookies

Ingredients

1 cup unsalted butter
1 cup crunchy peanut butter
1 cup white sugar
1 cup packed brown sugar
2 eggs
2 1/2 cups all-purpose flour
1 teaspoon baking powder
1/2 teaspoon salt
1 1/2 teaspoons baking soda

Directions

Cream together butter, peanut butter and sugars. Beat in eggs.

In a separate bowl, sift together flour, baking powder, baking soda, and salt. Stir into batter. Put batter in refrigerator for 1 hour.

Roll into 1 inch balls and put on baking sheets. Flatten each ball with a fork, making   a criss-cross pattern. Bake in a preheated 375 degrees F oven for about 10 minutes or until cookies begin to brown. Do not over-bake.

Peanut Butter Oatmeal Cookies II

Ingredients

2 cups white sugar
1/2 cup evaporated milk
1/4 cup unsweetened cocoa powder
1/2 cup butter
1/2 cup peanut butter
2 cups rolled oats

Directions

In a medium saucepan, put together the sugar, evaporated milk, cocoa powder, and butter; bring to a boil while stirring. Boil for 1 minute; remove from heat. Stir in the peanut butter and rolled oats. Drop by heaping teaspoonfuls onto waxed paper. Cool and serve.

Peanut Butter Puffs

Ingredients

3 tablespoons peanut butter
20 vanilla wafers
80 miniature marshmallows

Directions

Spread about 1/2 teaspoon peanut butter on each wafer. Place on a foil-lined baking sheet. Top each with four marshmallows. Broil for 2 -3 minutes or until the marshmallow are lightly browned. Serve warm.

Elvis Sandwich

Ingredients

3 tablespoons peanut butter
2 slices white bread
1 banana, peeled and sliced
3 slices cooked bacon
1 1/2 teaspoons butter

Directions

Spread the peanut butter on one side of one slice of bread. Top with sliced banana, then slices of cooked bacon. Cover with the other slice of bread. Spread butter on the outside of the sandwich.

Heat a skillet over medium heat. Fry the sandwich on each side until golden brown and peanut butter is melted, about 4 minutes total.

Peanut Butter Crispies II

Ingredients

6 cups crisp rice cereal
1 cup white sugar
1 cup peanut butter
1 cup corn syrup
1 tablespoon butter

Directions

In a medium sauce pan, mix together sugar, peanut butter, and corn syrup. Be careful not to let it burn, or it will ruin the recipe. Stir mixture until well melted. Remove pan from heat.

Combine warm peanut butter mixture with crisp rice cereal.

Grease well a 9 x 13 inch pan with butter or margarine. Spread mixture in pan. Allow to cool. When mixture is no longer sticky to the touch, cut into bars.

Easy Vegan Peanut Butter Fudge

Ingredients

3/4 cup vegan margarine
1 cup peanut butter
3 2/3 cups confectioners' sugar

Directions

Lightly grease a 9x9 inch baking dish.

In a saucepan over low heat, melt margarine. Remove from heat and stir in peanut butter until smooth. Stir in confectioners' sugar, a little at a time, until well blended. Pat into prepared pan and chill until firm. Cut into squares.

Easy Cake Mix Peanut Butter Cookies

Ingredients

1/4 cup butter
1/2 cup packed brown sugar
1 egg
1 (18 ounce) jar crunchy peanut butter
1 (18.25 ounce) package yellow cake mix

Directions

Preheat an oven to 350 degrees F (175 degrees C).

Beat the butter and sugar with an electric mixer in a large bowl until smooth. Add the egg and beat until incorporated; then beat in the peanut butter until evenly mixed. Stir in the cake mix until just incorporated. Shape the dough into 1 inch balls, place onto ungreased baking sheets, and flatten with a fork.

Bake in the preheated oven until the edges are golden, about 10 minutes. Allow the cookies to cool on the baking sheet for 1 minute before removing to a wire rack to cool completely.

Chocolate Peanut Butter Pie I

Ingredients

1 (9 inch) prepared chocolate cookie crumb crust
4 eggs
1 cup butter, softened
8 (1 ounce) squares semisweet chocolate
2 cups confectioners' sugar
1 cup smooth peanut butter
1/3 cup heavy whipping cream

Directions

Melt 6 ounces semi sweet chocolate, and cool to room temperature. Beat the eggs with 3/4 cup butter or margarine, chocolate and confectioners' sugar for a FULL 5 minutes. Mixture will be thick and smooth.

In a separate bowl, beat the peanut butter, 1/4 cup butter, and cream.

Spoon chocolate filling into crust. Swirl peanut butter filling into chocolate filling.

Drizzle remaining 2 oz of melted chocolate on top of pie. Refrigerate for at least 1 hour, and serve.

Chocolate Peanut Butter Marble Cake

Ingredients

1/4 cup unsweetened cocoa powder
2 tablespoons confectioners' sugar
2 tablespoons butter, softened
2 tablespoons hot water
1 cup peanut butter chips
1 tablespoon shortening
1 (18.25 ounce) package white cake mix
1/2 cup packed brown sugar
1 1/4 cups water
3 eggs

Directions

Preheat oven to 350 degrees F (175 degrees C). With a non-stick cooking spray, coat a 13X9X2 inch baking pan. Dust with flour and set aside.

In a small bowl, stir together the cocoa, confectioners' sugar, butter and 2 tablespoons hot water until smooth and set aside.

In microwavable bowl, place peanut butter chips and shortening. Microwave on high for 1 minute, or until chips are melted and smooth when stirred.

In large bowl, combine cake mix, brown sugar, 1-1/4 cups water, eggs and reserved melted peanut butter mixture; beat on low speed of electric mixer until moistened. Increase speed to medium, beat 2 minutes until smooth. Remove 1-1/2 cups of the batter and add it to the reserved cocoa mixture; blend well.

Pour the peanut butter flavored batter into the prepared pan. Drop spoonfuls of the chocolate batter on top. Swirl with a knife or spatula for a marbled effect.

Bake at 350 degree F (175 degrees C) for 40 to 45 minutes or until a wooden toothpick inserted in the center comes out clean. Cool and frost as desired.

EAGLE BRAND® Frozen Peanut Butter Pie

Ingredients

Chocolate Crunch Crust:
1/3 cup butter or margarine
1 (6 ounce) package semi-sweet chocolate chips
2 1/2 cups oven-toasted rice cereal

Pie filling:
1 (8 ounce) package cream cheese, softened
1 (14 ounce) can EAGLE BRAND® Sweetened Condensed Milk
3/4 cup Jif® Creamy Peanut Butter
2 tablespoons lemon juice
1 teaspoon vanilla extract
1 cup whipping cream, whipped
Smucker's® Chocolate Fudge Spoonable Ice Cream Topping

Directions

Chocolate Crunch Crust: In heavy saucepan, over low heat, melt butter or margarine and semi-sweet chocolate chips. Remove from heat; gently stir in oven-toasted rice cereal until completely coated. Press on bottom and up side to rim of buttered 9-inch or 10-inch pie plate. Chill 30 minutes.

Pie filling: In large bowl, beat cream cheese until fluffy; gradually beat in sweetened condensed milk then peanut butter until smooth.

Stir in lemon juice and vanilla. Fold in whipped cream. Turn into prepared crust.

Drizzle topping over pie. Freeze 4 hours or until firm. Return leftovers to freezer.

Peanut Butter Oatmeal Cookies

Ingredients

3 egg whites
1 cup packed brown sugar
1 cup reduced fat peanut butter
1/2 cup unsweetened applesauce
1/4 cup honey
2 teaspoons vanilla extract
3 cups quick-cooking oats
1 cup all-purpose flour
1 cup nonfat dry milk powder
2 teaspoons baking soda

Directions

In a mixing bowl, beat egg whites and brown sugar. Beat in peanut butter, applesauce, honey and vanilla. Combine the oats, flour, milk powder and baking soda; gradually add to peanut butter mixture, beating until combined.

Drop by tablespoonfuls 2 in. apart onto baking sheets coated with nonstick cooking spray. Bake at 350 degrees F for 8-10 minutes or until golden brown. Remove to wire racks to cool.

Ingredients

2 cups creamy peanut butter
1/2 cup butter
4 cups confectioners' sugar
3 cups crisp rice cereal
2 cups semisweet chocolate chips

Directions

Melt peanut butter and butter in saucepan, over low heat. In large bowl, mix crispy rice cereal and confectioners' sugar well. Pour melted peanut butter and butter over cereal and sugar and blend together thoroughly.

Form into 1 inch or smaller balls, spread on cookie sheets, chill till firm in refrigerator (over night is okay).

Melt chocolate in double boiler and keep melted while working with balls. A teaspoon is best to use in dipping the balls in chocolate. Dip good and place on cookie sheet. As you dip them place them back on cookie sheet and keep chilled till firm.

Double Layer Chocolate Peanut Butter Pie

Ingredients

1/2 (8 ounce) package cream cheese, softened
1 tablespoon white sugar
1 tablespoon cold milk
1 cup peanut butter
1 (8 ounce) container frozen whipped topping, thawed
1 (9 inch) prepared graham cracker crust
2 (3.9 ounce) packages instant chocolate pudding mix
2 cups cold milk
4 peanut butter cups, cut into 1/2 inch pieces

Directions

In a large bowl, mix cream cheese, sugar, 1 tablespoon milk and peanut butter until smooth. Gently stir in 1 1/2 cups of whipped topping. Spread mixture on bottom of pie crust.

In a second bowl, stir pudding mix with 2 cups milk until thick. Immediately stir in remaining whipped topping. Spread mixture over peanut butter layer.

Scatter peanut butter cups over top of pie. Cover and refrigerate for 4 hours.

Peanut Butter Drops

Ingredients

1 cup shortening
1 cup chunky peanut butter
1 cup packed brown sugar
1/2 cup sugar
2 eggs
1 teaspoon vanilla extract
1 cup shredded peeled zucchini
3 cups all-purpose flour
1 teaspoon salt
1/2 teaspoon baking powder
1/2 teaspoon baking soda

Directions

In a mixing bowl, cream the shortening, peanut butter and sugar. Beat in eggs and vanilla. Stir in zucchini. Combine dry ingredients; add to the zucchini mixture. Drop by rounded tablespoonfuls 2 in. apart onto greased baking sheet. Bake at 350 degrees F for 12-15 minutes or until lightly browned. Cool on wire racks.

Winter Peanut Snack Mix

Ingredients

1/4 cup butter
1/4 cup Jif® Creamy Peanut Butter & Honey
1/2 teaspoon vanilla extract
1 teaspoon ground cinnamon
4 cups honey and nut flavor checked cereal
1 cup honey roasted peanuts
1 cup pretzels (like midgets or snaps)
1/2 cup sunflower kernels
1 (6 ounce) package dried cranberries

Directions

Preheat oven to 350 degrees F.

Combine butter, peanut butter, vanilla extract and cinnamon in a microwave-safe bowl. Microwave on HIGH (100 percent power) 35 to 40 seconds; stir until well blended.

Combine cereal, peanuts, pretzels, sunflower kernels and cranberries in a large bowl.

Pour butter mixture over cereal mixture; toss well to coat.

Line sheet pan with foil; spread mixture evenly across pan. Bake 8 to 10 minutes, stirring occasionally; cool.

Store in resealable plastic bag.

Ham and Pumpkin Satay

Ingredients

2/3 cup peeled, cubed pumpkin
2/3 cup orange juice
1 1/2 tablespoons butter
1 onion, finely chopped
1 clove garlic, crushed
1 Thai or Serrano chile, chopped
1 teaspoon ground turmeric
1 teaspoon ground cumin
1 teaspoon ground nutmeg
1 teaspoon ground coriander seed
1 1/2 cups cooked, diced ham
2/3 cup crunchy peanut butter

Directions

Place the cubed pumpkin and orange juice in a small saucepan and bring it to a boil over medium-low heat. Simmer the pumpkin for 10 to 15 minutes, until it is soft. Carefully transfer to a blender, in batches if necessary, and blend until smooth.

Melt the butter in a skillet over medium heat, and cook and stir the onion, garlic, chile, turmeric, cumin, nutmeg, and coriander for 1 to 2 minutes. Stir in the ham, and cook and stir for about 5 minutes, until the ham has started to brown.

Pour the pureed pumpkin mixture into the spicy ham mixture, and stir the peanut butter into the sauce. Mix well to combine, and bring back to a simmer. Serve hot.

Peanut Butter Balls I

Ingredients

4 tablespoons butter
2 cups confectioners' sugar
1 cup shredded coconut
1 cup chopped walnuts
2/3 cup peanut butter
1/2 cup maraschino cherries, chopped
2 1/4 cups semisweet chocolate chips
1 cup flaked coconut

Directions

Melt butter or margarine over low heat. Remove from heat and mix melted butter, confectioners' sugar, coconut, walnuts, peanut butter and cherries. Form into small balls. Chill until firm.

Melt chocolate chips over low heat. Stick a toothpick into each ball and dip into chocolate. Roll chocolate covered peanut butter balls in coconut to coat. Chill.

Sugar-Free Peanut Butter Cookies

Ingredients

2 cups smooth natural peanut butter
2 cups granular no-calorie sucralose sweetener (e.g., Splenda ®)
2 large eggs

Directions

Preheat oven to 350 degrees F (175 degrees C). Lightly grease a baking sheet.

Thoroughly mix together the peanut butter, sucralose, and eggs in a bowl. Drop mixture by spoonfuls onto the prepared baking sheet.

Bake in the preheated oven until center appears dry, about 8 minutes.

Tried 'n' True Peanut Butter Cookies

Ingredients

4 cups butter flavored shortening
4 cups peanut butter
3 cups sugar
3 cups packed brown sugar
8 eggs
4 teaspoons vanilla extract
2 teaspoons water
9 cups all-purpose flour
4 teaspoons baking soda
4 teaspoons salt

Directions

In a large mixing bowl, cream shortening, peanut butter and sugars. Add eggs, one at a time, beating well after each addition. Beat in vanilla and water. Combine flour, baking soda and salt; gradually add to the creamed mixture.

Drop by heaping tablespoons 2 in. apart onto ungreased baking sheets. Flatten with a fork. Bake at 350 degrees F for 12-15 minutes or until golden brown. Remove to wire racks to cool.

Chewy Peanut Butter Crisps

Ingredients

1 cup peanut butter
1 cup sugar
1/2 cup evaporated milk
4 teaspoons cornstarch
1/2 cup semisweet chocolate chips

Directions

In a mixing bowl, combine peanut butter and sugar. Stir in milk and cornstarch until smooth. Add chocolate chips.

Drop by heaping teaspoonfuls 2 in. apart onto ungreased baking sheets. Bake at 350 degrees F for 12-15 minutes or until golden brown. Remove to wire racks to cool.

Peanut Butter Cup Grilled Sandwich

Ingredients

2 teaspoons margarine
2 slices white bread
1 1/2 tablespoons peanut butter
2 tablespoons semisweet chocolate chips

Directions

Spread 1 teaspoon of margarine onto one side of each slice of bread. Put the margarine sides together. This is to keep from getting margarine on your hands when spreading peanut butter. Spread peanut butter over one slice of bread, and sprinkle chocolate chips onto the peanut butter. Remove the other slice of bread from the back of the peanut butter slice, and place margarine side out over the peanut butter and chocolate chips.

Place a skillet over medium heat. Fry sandwich until golden brown on each side, 2 to 3 minutes. Cool slightly before cutting in half.

Caramel Nougat Bar Peanut Butter Cookies

Ingredients

1/2 cup white sugar
1/2 cup packed brown sugar
1/2 cup butter
1 teaspoon vanilla extract
1/2 cup peanut butter
1 egg
1 1/2 cups all-purpose flour
1/2 teaspoon baking soda 1/2 teaspoon baking powder 1/4 teaspoon salt
36 fun size bars milk chocolate covered caramel and nougat candy

Directions

Cream together white sugar, brown sugar, butter or margarine, vanilla, peanut butter and the egg.

Add in flour, baking soda, baking powder, and salt.

Wrap 1 heaping teaspoon of dough around a bite sized milk chocolate covered caramel and nougat candy bar. Bake 13-16 minutes at 350 degrees F (175 degrees C). Let cool 5 minutes before removing from pan.

Sheryl's Corn and Crab Chowder

Ingredients

5 slices bacon
1 tablespoon clarified butter
3/4 cup chopped onion
1/4 cup chopped green bell pepper
1/2 cup chopped celery
1 1/2 teaspoons minced garlic

1/4 cup dry white wine
1 teaspoon brandy
1 1/2 teaspoons dried basil
1 teaspoon ground white pepper
1/4 teaspoon cayenne pepper
1/2 teaspoon dried thyme leaves
2 teaspoons Worcestershire sauce
3 cups fresh corn kernels
4 large potatoes, peeled and diced
1 1/2 quarts chicken stock
1/2 cup butter
1/2 cup all-purpose flour

3 cups heavy cream
1 cup half-and-half cream
1 pound peeled and deveined small shrimp
1 tablespoon Creole seasoning
1 pound fresh lump crabmeat, shell pieces removed

Directions

Place the bacon in a large, deep skillet, and cook over medium-high heat, turning occasionally, until evenly browned, about 10 minutes. Remove the bacon, and reserve the grease. Allow the bacon to cool, then crumble, and set aside with the grease.

Meanwhile, heat 1 tablespoon of clarified butter in a large pot over medium heat. Stir in the onion, green pepper, celery, and garlic. Cook and stir until the onion has softened and turned translucent, about 10 minutes. Pour in the white wine and brandy, and bring to a simmer. Season with the basil, white pepper, cayenne pepper, thyme, and Worcestershire sauce. Add the corn and potatoes, then pour in the chicken stock. Bring to a boil over high heat, then reduce heat to medium-low, cover, and simmer 10 minutes.

While the soup is simmering, melt 1/2 cup of butter in a small saucepan over medium-low heat. Stir in the flour, and cook, stirring constantly, until the flour has turned the color of peanut butter to make a roux, about 10 minutes.

Stir the roux into the soup, and pour in the heavy cream, half-and-half cream, reserved bacon and grease, and shrimp. Return to a simmer over medium-high heat, and cook until the shrimp are no longer translucent in the center, the potatoes are tender, and the soup has thickened, about 15 minutes. Season to taste with Creole seasoning, and stir in the crab meat to serve.

Ground Nut Stew

Ingredients

2 cups peanut butter
1/2 (6 ounce) can tomato paste
2 (10 ounce) cans diced tomatoes with green chile peppers
4 cups chicken broth
2 tablespoons vegetable oil
6 skinless, boneless chicken breast halves - cubed
1 onion, chopped
1/2 cup fresh mushrooms, sliced
cayenne pepper to taste

Directions

Melt peanut butter in a large saucepan over medium heat. Stir in tomato paste, and blend with peanut butter until smooth. Mix in diced tomatoes with green chile peppers and chicken broth. Cook 15 minutes, stirring occasionally.

Heat oil in a medium skillet over medium heat. Saute chicken and onions until chicken is no longer pink and juices run clear.

Mix chicken, onions, and mushrooms into the peanut butter mixture, and continue cooking, stirring occasionally, about 15 minutes. Season with cayenne pepper.

No-Bake Peanut Butter Squares

Ingredients

1 cup JIF® Creamy Peanut Butter
1/2 teaspoon almond extract
1/4 cup butter, softened
1 1/4 cups sifted powdered sugar
2 cups crisp rice cereal
1/2 cup coarsely chopped peanuts

Directions

Line an 8-inch square baking pan with aluminum foil, extending foil over edges of pan. Blend peanut butter, almond extract and butter in large bowl; stir in powdered sugar. Add cereal; mix well, crushing cereal slightly.

Press peanut butter mixture evenly into prepared pan with rubber spatula. Sprinkle top with chopped peanuts; press gently. Chill. To serve, remove from pan by lifting foil; remove foil. Cut into 1-inch squares.

Peanut Butter Pie IX

Ingredients

1 (20 ounce) package chocolate sandwich cookies
1/2 cup butter, melted
2 (8 ounce) packages cream cheese, softened
2 cups white sugar
2 (16 ounce) jars crunchy peanut butter
1 (16 ounce) package frozen whipped topping, thawed
1/8 cup grated semisweet chocolate

Directions

In a food processor grind the cookies. Mix with the melted butter. Place into two pie pans and freeze.

Whip the cream cheese and slowly add sugar. Mix for 3 minutes on high speed. Add the peanut butter and mix. On low speed, mix in the whipped topping. Divide in two and place in pie pans lined with cookie crust.

Let set overnight in the freezer or in refrigerator. Garnish with whipped cream and shaved chocolate.

Cocoa Strawberry Pie

Ingredients

1/4 cup peanut butter
1/4 cup light corn syrup
2 cups Kellogg's® Cocoa Krispies® cereal
1 quart strawberry-flavored frozen yogurt or ice cream softened
Chocolate syrup (optional)
Sliced strawberries for garnish (optional)

Directions

In medium-size mixing bowl, stir together peanut butter and corn syrup. Add Kellogg's® Cocoa Krispies® cereal. Stir until well coated. Press evenly on bottom and side of 9-inch pie pan. Chill in refrigerator about 15 minutes.

Spoon frozen yogurt into crust. Freeze until firm, about 3 hours. Remove from freezer 10 minutes before serving. Drizzle chocolate syrup on top and garnish with sliced strawberries, if desired.

EZ Peanut Butter Pie II

Ingredients

1 (9 inch) prepared graham cracker crust
1 (4.6 ounce) package non-instant vanilla pudding mix
1 cup peanut butter

Directions

Prepare cook and serve pudding as directed on package. Stir in peanut butter. Bring mixture to a boil and pour into graham cracker crust. Allow to cool.

World's Best Peanut Butter Fudge

Ingredients

4 cups white sugar
1 cup milk
1/2 cup butter
1 (7 ounce) jar marshmallow creme
12 ounces peanut butter
2/3 cup all-purpose flour

Directions

Grease a 9x13 inch baking dish, set aside.

In a saucepan, combine sugar, milk, and butter. Bring to a boil, and cook 5 minutes. Remove from the heat. Stir in the marshmallow creme and peanut butter. Gradually stir in the flour. Spread into the prepared pan, and let cool.

Jif® Peanut Butter Fudge

Ingredients

Crisco® Original No-Stick Cooking Spray
3 cups granulated sugar
1/2 cup butter or margarine
2/3 cup PET® Evaporated Milk
1 2/3 cups Jif® Creamy Reduced Fat Peanut Spread
1 (7 ounce) jar marshmallow creme
1 teaspoon vanilla

Directions

Line a 13 x 9 x 2-inch pan with aluminum foil and then spray with a no-stick cooking spray.

Combine sugar, butter and milk in large saucepan, stirring constantly on medium heat, until mixture comes to a boil.

Boil 5 minutes, stirring constantly. Remove from heat.

Add peanut butter. Stir until well blended. Add marshmallow creme and vanilla. Beat until well blended.

Spread in prepared pan. Cool.

Cut into candy-sized pieces. Store in covered container.

Winter Energy Cookies

Ingredients

1 cup unsalted butter
1 1/2 cups packed brown sugar
1/3 cup molasses
1/3 cup smooth peanut butter
2 eggs
1 1/2 teaspoons vanilla extract
1 1/2 cups whole wheat flour
1 cup all-purpose flour
1 cup toasted wheat germ
1 1/2 teaspoons baking soda
1/2 teaspoon salt
1/2 teaspoon ground cinnamon
2 cups rolled oats
1 cup raisins
1 cup semisweet chocolate chips
1 cup chopped walnuts

Directions

Cream the butter, sugar, molasses, and peanut butter in a large bowl. Blend in the eggs and vanilla. Mix the flour, wheat germ, baking soda, salt, and cinnamon in a separate bowl. Stir the dry ingredients into the creamed mixture, until evenly blended.

Stir in the oats, raisins, choc chips, and nuts. Cover and refrigerate for 1 hour.

Preheat oven to 350 degrees F (180 degrees C).

Shape dough into large balls using 1/4 cup of dough per cookie. Place on greased cookie sheets, leaving 3 inches between them. Flatten slightly with a fork. Bake for 15 to 18 minutes. When done, the tops will still be soft to the touch. Cool on the sheets for 5 minutes, then transfer to a rack to cool.

Peanut Butter Berry Delights

Ingredients

1/2 cup creamy peanut butter
5 tablespoons milk chocolate chips, melted and cooled
2 tablespoons whipped topping
20 large fresh strawberries
5 (1 ounce) squares semisweet chocolate, melted

Directions

Line a baking sheet with waxed paper; set aside. In a small bowl, combine the peanut butter, melted milk chocolate and whipped topping.

Beginning at the right of the stem, cut each strawberry in half diagonally. Scoop out the white portion from the larger half of each berry. Spread or pipe peanut butter mixture between the two halves; press gently. Place on prepared pan; refrigerate for 15 minutes or until set. Dip bottom half of berries in semisweet chocolate. Place on pan. Refrigerate for 15-20 minutes or until set.

Doubly Delicious Peanut Butter Cookies

Ingredients

1 cup white sugar
1 cup packed brown sugar
1 cup crunchy peanut butter
1/2 cup butter flavored shortening
2 eggs
1 1/2 cups all-purpose flour
1/2 teaspoon baking soda
1/4 teaspoon salt
2 cups peanut butter chips

Directions

Preheat oven to 350 degrees F (175 degrees C).

Combine sugars, peanut butter and shortening in large bowl. Beat at medium speed of mixer until well blended. Add eggs, one at a time, beating well afer each addition. Combine flour, baking soda and salt. Add gradually to creamed mixture at low speed. Mix just until blended. Stir in peanut butter chips with spoon. (Dough will be stiff.)

Shape into 1 1/2 inch balls. Place 2 inches apart on ungreased baking sheet. Make crisscross marks on top with floured fork tines.

Bake for 8 to 10 minutes or until edges are set and tops are moist. Cool about 8 minutes on baking sheet before removing to flat surface.

Nigerian Peanut Soup

Ingredients

4 cups chicken broth
1 jalapeno pepper, seeded and minced
1/2 cup chopped green bell pepper
1/2 cup chopped onion
1/2 cup crunchy peanut butter

Directions

In 1-quart saucepan add broth and chili peppers and bring mixture to a boil. Stir in bell pepper and onion and return to a boil. Reduce heat to low, cover, and let simmer until vegetables are tender, about 10 minutes.

Reduce heat to lowest possible temperature; add peanut butter and cook, stirring constantly, until peanut butter is melted and mixture is well blended.

'King Of Rock' Frozen Pudding Pops

Ingredients

2 cups cold milk
1 (3.5 ounce) package instant banana pudding mix
1 1/2 teaspoons warm peanut butter

Directions

Pour the cold milk into a large bowl; whisk the pudding mix into the cold milk until dissolved, about 2 minutes. Allow to rest until nearly set, 4 to 5 minutes.

Mash the peanut butter into the pudding; stir to distribute the peanut butter evenly throughout the mixture. Spoon the mixture into popsicle molds, tapping the mold on a hard surface to allow any air bubbles to escape. Store in freezer until completely frozen solid, 5 hours to overnight. Running warm water over the outside of the mold will make it easier to remove the pops.

Peanut Butter Heaven

Ingredients

1 cup butter, softened
1 cup white sugar
1 cup brown sugar
2 eggs
3/4 cup peanut butter
2 cups rolled oats
2 cups all-purpose flour
1 teaspoon baking soda
2 1/2 cups semisweet chocolate chips
1/2 cup peanut butter

Directions

Preheat oven to 350 degrees F (175 degrees C). Grease a 9x13 inch baking pan.

In a large bowl, cream together the butter, white sugar and brown sugar. Beat in the eggs, one at a time, then stir in the 3/4 cup peanut butter. Combine the oats, flour and baking soda; stir into the creamed mixture until well blended. Press the dough evenly into the prepared pan.

Bake for 15 to 20 minutes in the preheated oven, until firm. In the microwave or over a double boiler, melt chocolate chips and 1/2 cup peanut butter together, stirring frequently until smooth. Spread over cooled bars and allow to set up before cutting into squares.

Protein Popcorn

Ingredients

1/3 cup light corn syrup
1/3 cup honey
1/3 cup white sugar
3/4 cup peanut butter
1 teaspoon vanilla extract
3 (3.5 ounce) packages microwave popcorn, popped

Directions

Bring the corn syrup, honey, and sugar to a boil in a saucepan; cook at a boil for 2 minutes. Immediately remove from heat and stir the peanut butter and vanilla into the syrup mixture until the peanut butter has melted completely.

Pour the popcorn into a large bowl; pour the sauce over the popcorn and stir until evenly coated. Allow to cool completely and break into chunks to serve.

Peanut Butter Fudgy Bars

Ingredients

Crisco® Original No-Stick
Cooking Spray
1 (18.25 ounce) package
Pillsbury® Golden Butter Cake
1 cup JIF® Extra Crunchy Peanut
Butter
1/2 cup water
1 large egg
1 (16 ounce) container Pillsbury®
Chocolate Fudge Frosting
1/2 cup Jif® Extra Crunchy
Peanut Butter
1/2 cup candy-coated chocolate
pieces
1/2 cup chopped peanuts

Directions

Heat oven to 350 degrees F. Lightly spray 13 x 9-inch pan with no-stick cooking spray. In large bowl, combine cake mix, 1 cup peanut butter, water and egg on low speed, mixing 2 minutes on medium speed. Spread into prepared pan.

Bake at 350 degrees F for 20 to 25 minutes or until puffed and light golden brown. Cool completely.

Blend frosting with 1/2 cup peanut butter in a small bowl. Spread over cooled bars.

Top with candy pieces and chopped peanuts.

Peanut Butter Cake II

2 cup creamy peanut butter
2 cup butter, softened
eggs
(18.25 ounce) package butter
ake mix
3 cup water

cup peanut butter
2 cup butter, softened
cups confectioners' sugar
3 cup heavy cream

Directions

Preheat oven to 325 degrees F (165 degrees C). Grease and flour two 9 inch round cake pans.

Combine 1/2 cup peanut butter and 1/2 cup butter or margarine. Cream until light and fluffy. Add eggs one at time, mixing well after each one. Add cake mix alternately with the water. Stir until just combined. Pour batter into prepared pans.

Bake at 325 degrees F (165 degrees C) for 25 minutes or until cake tests done. Allow cakes to cool in pan for 10 minutes and then turn out onto a cooling rack to cool completely. Assemble and frost with Peanut Butter Frosting once cool.

To Make Peanut Butter Frosting: Combine 1 cup peanut butter, and 1/2 cup butter or margarine cream together until light and fluffy. Add the confectioner's sugar. Mix in enough cream to make the frosting of a spreading consistency. Apply to cool cake.

Ginger-Touched Oatmeal Peanut Butter Cookies

Ingredients

1/2 cup butter
1/2 cup shortening
1 cup peanut butter
1 cup packed brown sugar
3/4 cup white sugar
2 eggs
1/2 teaspoon vanilla extract
1 1/2 cups all-purpose flour
2 teaspoons baking soda
1 teaspoon salt
1 teaspoon ground ginger
1 cup rolled oats
1 cup chopped crystallized ginger

Directions

Preheat oven to 350 degrees F (175 degrees C).

In a medium bowl, cream together the shortening, butter, brown sugar and white sugar. Beat in the eggs, peanut butter and vanilla. Combine the flour, baking soda, salt and ground ginger, stir into the creamed mixture. Finally, stir in the rolled oats and candied ginger. Drop by rounded teaspoonfuls onto an unprepared cookie sheet.

Bake for 10 to 12 minutes in the preheated oven, until golden brown. Remove from the baking sheet to cool on wire racks. Store in an airtight container when cool.

Peanut Butter Crunch Bars

Ingredients

3 3/4 cups powdered sugar
1/2 cup butter
1 (16 ounce) jar SMUCKER'S®
Natural Peanut Butter
3 cups crispy cereal or corn flakes
1 (16 ounce) package of semi-sweet chocolate chips

Directions

Melt butter over low heat in sauce pan.

In a mixing bowl, blend peanut butter and sugar. Add the melted butter and continue to blend.

Stir in cereal and spread evenly onto a 9 x 13-inch pan.

In a separate saucepan, melt the chocolate chips over low heat.

Spread melted chocolate evenly over bars. Refrigerate to cool. Cut into bars.

Coconut Granola Bars

Ingredients

3/4 cup packed brown sugar
2/3 cup peanut butter
1/2 cup corn syrup
1/2 cup butter or margarine, melted
2 teaspoons vanilla extract
3 cups old-fashioned oats
1 cup semisweet chocolate chips
1/2 cup flaked coconut
1/2 cup sunflower kernels
1/3 cup wheat germ
2 teaspoons sesame seeds

Directions

In a large bowl, combine brown sugar, peanut butter, corn syrup, butter and vanilla. Combine the remaining ingredients; add to peanut butter mixture and stir to coat. Press into two greased 13-in. x 9-in. x 2-in. baking pans. Bake at 350 degrees F for 25-30 minutes or until golden brown. Cool on wire racks. Cut into bars.

Peanut Butter Clusters

Ingredients

1 (10 ounce) package Reese's Peanut Butter Chips
1/2 cup dry-roasted unsalted peanuts
1/2 cup regular oats, uncooked
1/2 cup raisins
1 teaspoon cinnamon

Directions

Microwave chips in a bowl on high power until melted, about 1 1/2 minutes. Stir. Add remaining ingredients; mix thoroughly. Using your hands, firmly roll into 1-inch balls. Cool.

Spicy Peanut Chicken

Ingredients

1 1/2 teaspoons curry powder
2 tablespoons Thai chili garlic sauce (Sriracha), or to taste
1 1/2 teaspoons ground cayenne pepper, or to taste
1/2 teaspoon ground cinnamon
2 teaspoons soy sauce
1/2 pound uncooked spaghetti
1 tablespoon peanut oil
2 large skinless, boneless chicken breast halves, cut into 1-inch cubes
3 1/2 cups water
2 cups extra chunky peanut butter
4 green onions, coarsely chopped
1/2 cup chow mein noodles

Directions

Combine curry powder, Thai chili garlic sauce, cayenne pepper, cinnamon, and soy sauce in a small bowl, and set aside. Fill a saucepan with water, and bring it to a boil. When the water is boiling, drop in the spaghetti and cook for 8 to 12 minutes, stirring occasionally, until tender. Drain the spaghetti, and set aside.

Heat peanut oil in a skillet or wok over medium-high heat until barely smoking, and drop in the chicken. Cook and stir 5 to 8 minutes, until the chicken is just beginning to brown and the inside is no longer pink. Remove chicken from the skillet, and set aside.

Make the peanut sauce by stirring together peanut butter and 3 1/2 cups of water in a saucepan over medium heat until mixture is smooth and the peanut butter is melted. Pour in the curry-chili sauce, and simmer, stirring occasionally, until the sauce is thickened, about 15 minutes.

To serve, place the noodles in a large bowl, top with chicken, and spoon the peanut sauce over the chicken. Sprinkle the green onions over the dish, and garnish with chow mein noodles.

Oatmeal Peanut Butter Cookies

Ingredients

1/2 cup shortening
1/2 cup margarine, softened
1 cup packed brown sugar
3/4 cup white sugar
1 cup peanut butter
2 eggs
1 1/2 cups all-purpose flour
2 teaspoons baking soda
1 teaspoon salt
1 cup quick-cooking oats

Directions

Preheat oven to 350 degrees F (175 degrees C).

In a large bowl, cream together shortening, margarine, brown sugar, white sugar, and peanut butter until smooth. Beat in the eggs one at a time until well blended. Combine the flour, baking soda, and salt; stir into the creamed mixture. Mix in the oats until just combined. Drop by teaspoonfuls onto ungreased cookie sheets.

Bake for 10 to 15 minutes in the preheated oven, or until just light brown. Don't over-bake. Cool and store in an airtight container.

Nutty Buddy Pies

Ingredients

1 (8 ounce) package cream cheese, softened
1 cup milk
2 cups confectioners' sugar
2/3 cup crunchy peanut butter
2 cups frozen whipped topping, thawed
3 (9 inch) prepared graham cracker crusts
3/4 cup chocolate syrup
1 cup chopped salted peanuts

Directions

In a large bowl, beat the cream cheese and milk until blended. Mix in the sugar and peanut butter until smooth, then fold in the whipped topping.

Spoon mixture into all 3 graham cracker crusts. Drizzle each with chocolate syrup and a sprinkle of peanuts. Cover and freeze for about 2 to 3 hours.

Let stand 30 minutes at room temperature before serving.

Sparky's Doggie Treats

Ingredients

1 cup all-purpose flour
1 cup corn flour
1 cup cornmeal
1/2 cup smooth peanut butter
1 cup water
1/3 cup vegetable oil
1 egg

Directions

Preheat oven to 375 degrees F (190 degrees C). Whisk together the flour, corn flour, and cornmeal in a mixing bowl. Lightly grease two baking sheets.

Place the peanut butter in a microwave safe dish, and cook in the microwave a few seconds at a time until the peanut butter has liquefied. Stir the peanut butter, water, vegetable oil, and egg into the flour mixture until a stiff dough forms. Roll out on a floured surface and cut into treat shapes with a cookie cutter. Place the treats onto the prepared cookie sheets.

Bake in the preheated oven until golden, 10 to 12 minutes. Allow the treats to cool on the baking sheets for 5 minutes before removing to a wire rack to cool completely. Store in an airtight container.

Peanut Butter Granola

Ingredients

9 cups rolled oats
3/4 cup whole wheat flour
1 1/2 cups chopped walnuts
2 tablespoons brewers' yeast (optional)
1/2 teaspoon salt, or to taste
1 cup dry milk powder
1 cup shredded coconut

3/4 cup white sugar
1/2 cup water
3/4 cup canola oil
1 cup unsalted peanut butter

Directions

Preheat an oven to 300 degrees F (150 degrees C).

Combine the oats, flour, walnuts, yeast, salt, milk powder, and coconut in a large mixing bowl; set aside. Stir the sugar, water, canola oil, and peanut butter together in a small saucepan over low heat until the sugar has dissolved and the mixture is hot and smooth. Pour the peanut butter over the oats and stir until evenly combined. Spread out onto 4 baking sheets.

Bake in the preheated oven for 45 minutes, stirring every 15 minutes. Turn the oven off and allow the granola to cool in the oven until dry, about 3 hours.

Peanut Butter Glaze

Ingredients

4 teaspoons water
2/3 cup powdered sugar
1 tablespoon creamy peanut butter

Directions

Stir together the water, sugar, and peanut butter until smooth.

Dessert Nachos

Ingredients

1/3 cup peanut butter
2 tablespoons confectioners' sugar
1/2 cup chocolate chips
2 1/2 cups mini round corn tortilla chips
1/4 cup miniature marshmallows
1/4 cup sweetened flaked coconut

Directions

Preheat your oven's broiler.

Combine the peanut butter and confectioners' sugar in a microwave-safe bowl. Heat the mixture until the peanut butter melts, about 1 minute. Place the chocolate chips in a separate microwave-safe bowl; melt the chips in the microwave, about 1 minute.

Arrange the tortilla chips into an even layer on a baking sheet. Drizzle the peanut butter mixture and the melted chocolate over the chips. Scatter the marshmallows and coconut over the chips.

Place under preheated broiler until the marshmallows begin to brown, 2 to 3 minutes. Serve hot.

Card Club Dessert

Ingredients

2 1/4 cups crushed chocolate sandwich cookies

1/3 cup butter or margarine, melted

1 3/4 cups cold milk

1 (3.4 ounce) package instant vanilla pudding mix

1 cup peanut butter

1 (4 ounce) bar German sweet chocolate, chopped

1 (12 ounce) container frozen whipped topping, thawed

Directions

In a bowl, combine cookie crumbs and butter; set aside 1/4 cup for topping. Press remaining crumb mixture into an ungreased 13-in. x 9-in. x 2-in. baking pan. Bake at 375 degrees F for 5 minutes; cool completely. In a mixing bowl, beat milk and pudding mix for 2 minutes or until thickened. Immediately stir in peanut butter and chocolate. Fold in whipped topping. Spread over cooled crust. Sprinkle with reserved crumb mixture. Cover and refrigerate for 4 hours or overnight.

Nutty Butter Munchies

Ingredients

1 cup butter or margarine, softened
1/2 cup chunky peanut butter
1 cup sugar
1 cup packed brown sugar
3 eggs
1 teaspoon vanilla extract
1/2 teaspoon almond extract
3 cups all-purpose flour 1/2 teaspoon baking soda 1/2 teaspoon salt
1 1/2 cups chopped pecans
1/2 cup salted peanuts

Directions

In a mixing bowl, cream butter, peanut butter and sugars. Add eggs, one at a time, beating well after each addition. Beat in extracts. Combine flour, baking soda and salt; gradually add to the creamed mixture. Stir in nuts.

Drop by tablespoonfuls 2 in. apart onto greased baking sheets. Flatten with a glass dipped in sugar. Bake at 350 degrees F for 10 -12 minutes or until the edges are lightly browned. Remove to wire racks to cool.

Peanut Butter Pie VI

Ingredients

2/3 cup white sugar
1/3 cup peanut butter
1/2 cup white sugar
3 tablespoons cornstarch
1/2 teaspoon salt
2 cups milk
4 eggs, separated
1 (9 inch) pie shell, baked

Directions

Mix together 2/3 cup white sugar and peanut butter. Sprinkle 2/3 of the mixture into baked pie shell.

Combine 1/2 cup sugar, corn starch, salt, milk, and egg yolks in a medium saucepan. Cook and stir over medium low heat until thick. Pour filling over peanut butter mixture in pie shell.

In a clean glass bowl, beat egg whites until very stiff. Spread meringue on top of pie. Sprinkle remaining peanut butter crumbs on top of the egg whites.

Bake at 400 degrees F (205 degrees C) for 5 to 7 minutes, or until the meringue is golden brown.

Peanut Butter Cup Cookies II

Ingredients

1/2 cup butter
1/2 cup white sugar
1/2 cup packed brown sugar
1/2 cup peanut butter
1 egg
1/2 teaspoon vanilla extract
1 1/4 cups all-purpose flour
2/3 teaspoon baking soda
1/4 teaspoon salt
15 miniature chocolate covered peanut butter cups, unwrapped

Directions

Preheat oven to 350 degrees.

In a medium bowl, cream the butter, white sugar, brown sugar, and peanut butter together. Stir in the egg and vanilla. Sift together the flour, baking soda and salt; stir into the creamed mixture.

Drop by tablespoonfuls into the cups of a muffin tin. Cups should be about 1/4 full. Bake for 8 to 10 minutes, until lightly browned. Remove from oven and immediately press a peanut butter cup into the center of each cookie. Allow the cookies to cool completely before removing from their pan.

Tumbleweeds

Ingredients

1 (12 ounce) can salted peanuts
1 (7 ounce) can potato sticks
3 cups butterscotch chips
3 tablespoons peanut butter

Directions

Combine peanuts and potato sticks in a bowl; set aside. In a microwave, heat butterscotch chips and peanut butter at 70% power for 1-2 minutes or until melted, stirring every 30 seconds. Add to peanut mixture; stir to coat evenly. Drop by rounded tablespoonfuls onto waxed paper-lined baking sheets. Refrigerate until set, about 5 minutes. Store in an airtight container.

Peanut Butter Cookies with Chocolate Chunks

Ingredients

1 1/2 cups unbleached all-purpose flour
1/3 cup rolled oats
1 teaspoon baking soda
1/4 teaspoon salt
1 cup crunchy peanut butter
1 cup packed brown sugar
1/2 cup unsalted butter
1/4 cup honey
1 egg
1 teaspoon vanilla extract
5 (1 ounce) squares semisweet chocolate

Directions

Mix flour, oats, baking soda, and salt in medium bowl.

Using an electric mixer, beat peanut butter, brown sugar, butter, honey, egg, and vanilla in large bowl until well blended. Stir dry ingredients into the peanut butter mixture in 2 additions. Stir in chopped chocolate.

Cover and refrigerate until dough is firm and no longer sticky, about 30 minutes.

Preheat oven to 350 degrees F (175 degrees C). Butter 2 heavy large baking sheets.

With hands, roll 1 heaping tablespoonful of dough for each cookie into 1 3/4 inch diameter ball. Arrange cookies on prepared baking sheets, spacing 2 1/2 inches apart.

Bake cookies until puffed, beginning to brown on top and still very soft to touch, about 12 minutes. Cool cookies on baking sheets for 5 minutes. Using metal spatula, transfer cookies to rack and cool completely. (Can be made 2 days ahead. Store in airtight container at room temperature.)

Fudgy Pudding Treats

Ingredients

2 cups skim milk
1 (1 ounce) package sugar free fat free instant vanilla pudding mix
1/2 cup Smucker's® Sugar Free Hot Fudge Spoonable Ice Cream Topping
1/2 cup Smucker's® Chunky Natural Peanut Butter

Directions

Whisk together milk and pudding mix in medium bowl for 1 minute. Stir in hot fudge topping and peanut butter until smooth and creamy.

Pour 1/4 cup mixture into 12 small disposable plastic cups (4 or 5 oz. size). Insert a wooden stick in each treat.

Freeze 1 to 2 hours or until firm. Release treat by quickly running warm water on outside of cup.

No Bake Peanut Butter Pie

Ingredients

1 (8 ounce) package cream cheese
1 1/2 cups confectioners' sugar
1 cup peanut butter
1 cup milk
1 (16 ounce) package frozen whipped topping, thawed
2 (9 inch) prepared graham cracker crusts

Directions

Beat together cream cheese and confectioners' sugar. Mix in peanut butter and milk. Beat until smooth. Fold in whipped topping.

Spoon into two 9 inch graham cracker pie shells; cover, and freeze until firm.

Chocolate Chip Peanut Butter Blondies

Ingredients

1 cup margarine
2 cups white sugar
2 eggs
1 teaspoon vanilla extract
1 cup chunky peanut butter
2 cups all-purpose flour
1 teaspoon baking powder
2 cups semisweet chocolate chips

Directions

Preheat oven to 350 degrees F (175 degrees C). Line a 10x15 inch jellyroll pan with parchment paper.

In a medium bowl, cream together the margarine and sugar. Beat in the eggs, one at a time. Stir in the vanilla and peanut butter until smooth. Combine the flour and baking powder, then stir into the peanut butter mixture. Finally, fold in the chocolate chips. Spread the dough out flat on the prepared pan.

Bake for 12 to 15 minutes in the preheated oven, until the tops of the bars look dry. Cool in pan, then cut into squares.

Peanut Butter Pudding

Ingredients

1/3 cup sugar
4 1/2 teaspoons cornstarch
1/4 teaspoon salt
1 1/2 cups milk
1/2 cup half-and-half cream
1/2 cup creamy peanut butter
1 teaspoon vanilla extract
Whipped cream

Directions

In a saucepan, combine sugar, cornstarch and salt. Gradually stir in milk and cream; bring to a boil over medium heat. Cook and stir for 2 minutes. Remove from the heat; stir in peanut butter and vanilla until smooth. Pour into serving dishes; refrigerate. Garnish with whipped cream if desired.

Chocolate Peanut Butter Chip Cookies

Ingredients

2 1/2 cups all-purpose flour
1/2 teaspoon baking soda
1/4 teaspoon salt
1/2 cup unsweetened cocoa powder
1 cup butter, softened
1 cup packed brown sugar
3/4 cup white sugar
3 eggs
2 teaspoons vanilla extract
2 cups peanut butter chips

Directions

Preheat the oven to 300 degrees F (150 degrees C). In a small bowl, whisk together the flour, baking soda, salt and cocoa. Set aside.

In a large bowl, cream together the butter, brown sugar and white sugar until smooth. Beat in the eggs, one at a time, then stir in the vanilla. Gradually blend in the dry ingredients until just moistened, then stir in the peanut butter chips. Drop by rounded spoonfuls onto the prepared cookie sheet.

Bake for 18 to 20 minutes in the preheated oven. Remove cookies to cool on a wire rack.

Thai-Style Peanut Sauce

Ingredients

3 tablespoons brown sugar
2 tablespoons rice wine
2 teaspoons rice wine vinegar
1/4 cup coconut milk
3/4 cup peanut butter
1/4 teaspoon curry powder
2 teaspoons dark soy sauce
1/4 teaspoon toasted sesame oil
1/2 teaspoon minced garlic
1/2 teaspoon sweet chili sauce
1 teaspoon minced pickled ginger
1/2 teaspoon fish sauce

Directions

Mix together the brown sugar, rice wine, and rice wine vinegar in a small bowl until smooth.

Combine the coconut milk and peanut butter in a small saucepan over low heat. Heat and stir until the peanut butter melts, being careful to not allow the coconut milk to boil. Stir the sugar mixture into the coconut milk mixture; pour into a bowl; stir in the soy sauce, sesame oil, garlic, chili sauce, ginger, and fish sauce.

Brown Sugar Cookies II

Ingredients

2/3 cup shortening
2/3 cup butter, softened
1 cup white sugar
1 cup packed brown sugar
2 eggs
2 teaspoons vanilla extract
3 1/4 cups all-purpose flour
1 teaspoon baking soda
1 teaspoon salt

Directions

Mix shortening, butter or margarine, sugars, eggs and vanilla thoroughly. Stir in all purpose or unbleached flour, baking soda and salt.

Turn dough onto lightly floured board. Shape dough into ball with lightly floured hands, pressing to make dough compact. Cut dough in half.

Shape each half into a roll 2 inches in diameter and about 8 inches long by gently rolling dough back and forth on floured board. Roll dough onto plastic wrap: wrap and twist ends tightly. Dough can be refrigerated up to 1 month or frozen up to 3 months.

Preheat oven to 375 degrees F (190 degrees C).

Cut roll into 1/4-inch slices. (It is not necessary to thaw frozen dough before slicing.) Place slices about 2 inches apart on ungreased baking sheet. Bake 9 to 11 minutes. Immediately remove cookies from baking sheet onto wire rack.

CHOCOLATE CHIP: Add 1 cup mini semisweet chocolate chips and 1 cup chopped nuts with the flour. OATMEAL-COCONUT: Reduce flour to 2 3/4 cups. Add 1 cup flaked coconut and 1 cup quick-cooking oats with the flour. PEANUT BUTTER: Add 1 cup creamy or chunky peanut butter with the shortening. CHOCOLATE-NUT: Add 1 cup chopped nuts and 1/2 cup cocoa with the flour. FRUIT SLICES: Add 1 cup whole candied cherries, 1/2 cup chopped nuts and 1/2 cup cut-up mixed candied fruit with the flour.

Oatmeal Peanut Butter and Chocolate Chip

Ingredients

3/4 cup butter
1/2 cup white sugar
1 cup packed brown sugar
2 eggs
1/3 cup peanut butter
1/4 cup water
1 teaspoon vanilla extract
1 1/2 cups all-purpose flour
1/2 teaspoon baking soda
2 cups rolled oats
1 cup semisweet chocolate chips

Directions

Preheat oven to 350 degrees F (175 degrees C).

In a medium bowl, cream together the butter, brown sugar and white sugar. Beat in the eggs one at a time, then stir in the peanut butter, water and vanilla. Combine the flour and baking soda, stir into the creamed mixture. Finally, stir in the rolled oats and chocolate chips. Drop by teaspoonfuls onto an unprepared cookie sheet.

Bake for 8 to 10 minutes in the preheated oven, until the cookies are lightly toasted on the edges. Remove from the baking sheet to cool on wire racks.

Butterfinger Cookies

Ingredients

1/2 cup butter, softened
3/4 cup sugar
2/3 cup packed brown sugar
2 egg whites
1 1/4 cups chunky peanut butter
1 1/2 teaspoons vanilla extract
1 cup all-purpose flour
1/2 teaspoon baking soda
1/4 teaspoon salt
5 Butterfinger candy bars (2.1 ounces each), chopped

Directions

In a mixing bowl, cream butter and sugars. Add egg whites; beat well. Blend in peanut butter and vanilla. Combine flour, baking soda and salt; add to creamed mixture and mix well. Stir in candy bars. Shape into 1-1/2-in. balls and place on greased baking sheets. Bake at 350 degrees F for 10-12 minutes or until golden brown. Cool on wire racks.

Layered Chocolate and Peanut Butter Bars

Ingredients

Crisco® Original No-Stick Cooking Spray
1 cup semi-sweet chocolate chips
1 cup packed brown sugar
2/3 cup Jif® Creamy Peanut Butter
1/2 cup butter, softened
1 large egg
1 teaspoon vanilla extract 3/4 cup Pillsbury BEST® All Purpose Flour
1/2 teaspoon baking soda
1/2 teaspoon salt
1 1/2 cups quick rolled oats

Directions

Heat oven to 350 degrees F. Spray 13 x 9-inch pan with a no-stick cooking spray. Melt chocolate chips in dry, microwave-safe bowl on HIGH (100% power) 1 minute. Stir. Microwave at additional, 10- to 15-second intervals, stirring just until chips are melted. Set aside.

Beat together brown sugar, peanut butter and butter in large bowl with an electric mixer, until smooth and creamy. Add egg and vanilla. Beat until well blended.

Stir together flour, baking soda and salt. Add to peanut butter mixture. Beat just until combined. Stir in oats. Press 3/4 of dough into prepared baking pan. Spread evenly with melted chocolate. Dot chocolate layer with remaining dough.

Bake 24 to 26 minutes. Cool. Cut into 24 bars.

Marbled Peanut Butter Brownies

Ingredients

Crisco® Original No-Stick
Cooking Spray
2/3 cup Pillsbury BEST® All
Purpose Flour
1/2 teaspoon baking powder
1/4 teaspoon salt
3/4 cup firmly packed brown
sugar
3/4 cup Smucker's® Creamy
Natural Peanut Butter, stirred OR
Jif® Creamy Peanut Butter
1/4 cup butter, softened
2 large eggs
1 teaspoon vanilla extract 1/2
cup semisweet chocolate
chips, melted and cooled

Directions

Heat oven to 350 degrees F. Spray an 8 x 8-inch baking pan with no-stick cooking spray.

Combine flour, baking powder and salt in small bowl.

Combine brown sugar, peanut butter and butter in bowl of electric mixer. Beat until light and creamy. Add eggs and vanilla. Beat until fluffy. Stir in flour mixture just until blended. Spread in prepared pan.

Drizzle melted chocolate over batter. Using a small, sharp knife, swirl the chocolate into the top of the batter to create a marbled effect.

Bake 30 minutes or until toothpick inserted in center comes out clean. Cool in pan on cooling rack. Cut into 24 bars.

Peanut Butter Eggs II

Ingredients

2 cups creamy peanut butter
3/4 cup butter
3 1/2 cups confectioners' sugar
3 cups crispy rice cereal
1 (12 ounce) package semisweet chocolate chips
2 tablespoons shortening

Directions

In a mixing bowl, combine peanut butter and butter. Stir in confectioners' sugar and crisp rice cereal until a dough is formed. Place this mixture in the refrigerator for about an hour to allow it to cool until it is easier to work with. Shape mixture into egg shapes and freeze for 20 minutes.

Melt chocolate chips and shortening in a double boiler over low heat. When melted, dip egg shapes in chocolate. Place on waxed paper and allow to cool.

Grilled Peanut Butter Apple Sandwiches

Ingredients

1 Gala apple, peeled, cored, and thinly sliced
1/2 teaspoon white sugar
1/2 teaspoon ground cinnamon
8 tablespoons creamy peanut butter
8 slices whole wheat bread
1/4 cup unsalted butter

Directions

Mix cinnamon and sugar together in a small bowl. Spread one tablespoon of peanut butter onto one side of 8 slices of bread.

Arrange apple slices on 4 slices of bread. Sprinkle the cinnamon/sugar mixture evenly over the apples. Top with the remaining 4 slices of bread, peanut butter face down.

Melt the butter in a large skillet over medium heat. Fry sandwiches until browned, about 1 to 2 minutes on each side.

Raisin Peanut Butter Bran Cookies

Ingredients

1 cup whole wheat flour
1 teaspoon baking soda
1/2 cup peanut butter
1 cup butter
1 1/4 cups packed brown sugar
3/4 cup whole bran cereal
2 eggs
1 teaspoon vanilla extract
2 1/2 cups raisins
2 cups rolled oats

Directions

Preheat oven to 350 degrees F (175 degrees C). Line cookie sheets with aluminum foil or baking parchment.

In a large saucepan, melt the butter over medium heat. Add peanut butter and sugar and stir until melted. Remove from heat.

Transfer to large mixing bowl and stir in bran cereal. Stir in eggs and vanilla and mix well. Fold in raisins and oatmeal and stir until well blended.

Sift together flour and baking soda and add to mixture. Mix thoroughly.

Drop dough by tablespoonfuls onto cookie sheets. Dip a fork into water and press to flatten dough to 1/2 inch thickness.

Bake for 15 minutes, or until cookies are lightly colored. Reverse sheet once during baking time. Let stand on wire racks to cool.

Peanut Banana Muffins

Ingredients

1 1/2 cups all-purpose flour
1/2 cup sugar
1 teaspoon baking powder
1/2 teaspoon baking soda
1/2 teaspoon salt
1 egg
1/2 cup butter or margarine, melted
1 1/2 cups mashed ripe banana
3/4 cup peanut butter chips

Directions

In a bowl, combine the flour, sugar, baking powder, baking soda and salt. In another bowl, combine the egg, butter and bananas. Stir into dry ingredients just until moistened. Fold in chips. Fill greased or paper-lined muffin cups three-fourths full. Bake at 375 degrees F for 18-22 minutes or until toothpick comes out clean. Cool for 5 minutes before removing from pan to a wire rack.

Chocolate Chip Crispies

Ingredients

1 cup corn syrup
1 cup white sugar
1 1/2 cups peanut butter
8 cups crisp rice cereal
1 cup semisweet chocolate chips

Directions

Butter a 9x13 inch pan.

Pour the sugar, syrup, and peanut butter into a large microwave bowl. Microwave on high until it begins to bubble, two to three minutes. Once the mixture is boiling, remove from the microwave oven, and stir in the cereal and chocolate chips until coated.

Pour the mixture into the prepared pan. Wet hands, sling off the excess water, and press down the treats until smoothed. Let cool, and cut into squares.

Hockey Pucks

Ingredients

1 (16 ounce) jar peanut butter
1 (16 ounce) package buttery round crackers
1 pound semisweet chocolate, chopped

Directions

Spread 1 teaspoon peanut butter on a cracker and top with another cracker.

Place chocolate in top of double boiler; stir frequently over medium heat until melted.

Place cracker sandwiches onto a fork and dip into the chocolate. Drain excess chocolate and cool on waxed paper. Store in refrigerator or cover and freeze until ready to serve.

Peanut Butter Balls VII

Ingredients

1 cup peanut butter
1 cup honey
1 1/2 cups dry milk powder

Directions

In a medium bowl, stir together the peanut butter and honey. Add the powdered milk and mix until well blended. Roll into walnut sized balls and serve.

Sinfully Rich P 'n' B Pie

Ingredients

1 (8 ounce) package fat free cream cheese
1 (16 ounce) jar creamy peanut butter
3/4 cup honey
1 teaspoon vanilla extract
1 (8 ounce) container frozen whipped topping, thawed
1 cup peanut butter chips
1 (9 inch) prepared chocolate cookie crumb crust

Directions

In a large bowl, beat together cream cheese and peanut butter until well combined. Stir in honey and vanilla. Finally, fold in whipped topping and peanut butter chips.

Spoon whole mixture into pie crust, then allow to chill overnight.

Peanut Mallow Bars

Ingredients

1 (18.25 ounce) package yellow cake mix
2 tablespoons water
1/3 cup butter or margarine, softened
1 egg
4 cups miniature marshmallows

2 cups peanut butter chips
2/3 cup light corn syrup
1/4 cup butter or margarine
2 teaspoons vanilla extract
2 cups crisp rice cereal
2 cups salted peanuts

Directions

Preheat the oven to 350 degrees F (175 degrees C). Grease a 9x13 inch baking pan.

In a large bowl, mix together the cake mix, water, butter, and egg until well blended. Spread into the bottom of the prepared pan.

Bake for 20 minutes in the preheated oven, or until a toothpick inserted into the center comes out clean. Remove from the oven, and sprinkle the marshmallows over the top. Return to the oven for about 2 minutes, just to melt the marshmallows together. Remove from the oven, and place pan on a wire rack to cool.

In a saucepan, combine the peanut butter chips, corn syrup, and butter. Stir over medium-low heat until melted and well blended. Remove from the heat, and stir in the vanilla, rice cereal and peanuts. Spread in an even layer over the marshmallows. Allow the bars to cool completely before cutting into squares.

Peanut Butter Molasses Cookies

Ingredients

/4 cup butter, softened
/4 cup peanut butter 1/2
up white sugar
/4 cup honey
/4 cup unsulfured molasses
egg
teaspoon vanilla extract
 1/3 cups all-purpose flour
/2 teaspoon baking powder
/4 teaspoon baking soda 1/4
easpoon salt
/4 teaspoon ground nutmeg
 teaspoon ground cinnamon
/4 teaspoon ground ginger
/2 cup white sugar

Directions

Preheat the oven to 375 degrees F (190 degrees C). Grease cookie sheets.

In a medium bowl, cream together the butter, peanut butter and 1/2 cup white sugar until smooth. Stir in the honey, molasses, egg and vanilla. Combine the flour, baking powder, baking soda, salt, nutmeg, cinnamon and ginger. Stir the dry ingredients into the molasses mixture until well blended. Roll dough into walnut sized balls and roll the balls in the remaining 1/2 cup of sugar. Place cookies 2 inches apart onto the prepared cookie sheets. Press a criss cross into the top with a fork.

Bake for 8 to 10 minutes in the preheated oven. Cool on the baking sheet for 5 minutes before removing to wire racks to cool completely.

Easter Eggs

Ingredients

2 pounds confectioners' sugar
1/4 pound margarine, softened
1 (8 ounce) package cream cheese
2 teaspoons vanilla extract
12 ounces peanut butter
1 pound flaked coconut
4 cups semisweet chocolate chips
2 tablespoons shortening

Directions

In a mixing bowl, combine sugar, margarine, cream cheese and vanilla extract. Divide the batter in half and place each half of the batter in a bowl on its own. Stir peanut butter into one of the bowls and coconut into the second.

Using your hands, mold the dough into egg-shapes and arrange the forms on cookie sheets. Place the eggs in the freezer until frozen.

Once the eggs have frozen, melt the chocolate and shortening in the top of a double-boiler. Dip the eggs into the chocolate until coated. Place the eggs on wax paper lined cookie sheets and return to the freezer to harden. After the chocolate has hardened the eggs can be kept in the refrigerator.

Peanut Crunch Cake

Ingredients

1 (18.25 ounce) package yellow cake mix
1 cup peanut butter
1/2 cup packed brown sugar
1 cup water
3 eggs
1/4 cup vegetable oil
1 cup chopped peanuts
3/4 cup semisweet chocolate chips
3/4 cup peanut butter chips

Directions

Preheat oven to 350 degrees F (175 degrees C). Grease and flour one 13x9 inch pan.

In a mixing bowl beat cake mix, peanut butter, and brown sugar on low speed until crumbly. Set aside 1/2 cup of mixture. To the remainder add water, eggs, and oil, and beat on high for 2 minutes. Stir in 1/4 cup each of the chocolate chips and the peanut butter chips. Pour into prepared pan.

Combine peanuts, remainder of dough mix, and rest of the chips; sprinkle over batter.

Bake at 350 degrees F (175 degrees C) for 30 to 40 minutes. Cool completely.

Ingredients

3/4 cup white sugar
1/2 cup packed brown sugar
1 3/4 cups all-purpose flour
1 teaspoon baking powder
1/2 teaspoon baking soda
8 peanut butter cups, cut into 1/2 inch pieces

Directions

Mix together the flour, baking powder and baking soda. Set aside.

Layer ingredients in order given in a 1 quart "wide mouth" canning jar. Press each layer firmly in place. It will be a tight fit. Add chopped peanut butter cups last.

Attach these directions to Jar: Reese's Peanut Butter Cup Cookies   1. Remove peanut butter cups from jar. Set aside. 2. Empty remaining cookie mix into large mixing bowl. Use your hands to thoroughly blend mix.   3. Add 1/2 cup butter or margarine, softened at room temperature. DO NOT USE DIET MARGARINE. Add in 1 egg, slightly beaten, and 1 teaspoon vanilla. 4. Mix until completely blended. You will need to finish mixing with your hands. 5. Mix in peanut butter cups. 6. Shape into walnut sized balls. Place 2 inches apart on greased cookie sheets. 7. Bake at 375 degrees F (190 degrees C) for 12 to 14 minutes until edges are lightly browned. Cool 5 minutes on baking sheet. Remove cookies to racks to finish cooling. Makes 2 1/2 dozen cookies.

Chewy Whole Wheat Peanut Butter Brownies

Ingredients

1/3 cup margarine, softened
2/3 cup white sugar
1/2 cup packed brown sugar
2 eggs
1 cup peanut butter
1/2 teaspoon vanilla extract
2 tablespoons water
3/4 cup whole wheat flour
1/4 cup all-purpose flour
1/4 teaspoon salt
1 teaspoon baking powder
1/4 teaspoon baking soda

Directions

Preheat oven to 350 degrees F (175 degrees Celsius). Grease a 9x9 inch baking pan.

In a large mixing bowl, beat together margarine and sugars; add eggs one at a time, and beat until mixture is light and fluffy. Stir in peanut butter, vanilla, and water.

In a separate mixing bowl, mix together flours with salt, baking powder, and baking soda. Stir into peanut butter mixture and blend well. Spread batter into the prepared pan.

Bake in preheated oven for 30 to 35 minutes, or until the top springs back when touched. Cool and cut into 16 squares.

NILLA Chocolate Peanut Butter No-Bake Cake

Ingredients

1 cup cold milk
1/4 cup peanut butter
1 pkg. (4 serving size) JELL-O Chocolate Instant Pudding
1 1/2 cups thawed COOL WHIP Whipped Topping
55 NILLA Wafers, divided
2 squares BAKER'S Semi-Sweet Chocolate
2 cups whole strawberries

Directions

Add milk to peanut butter in medium bowl, beating with wire whisk until well blended. Add dry pudding mix. Beat 2 minutes or until well blended. Stir in the whipped topping.

Reserve 5 of the wafers for later use. Spread about 1 teaspoon of the pudding mixture onto each of the remaining 50 wafers. Stack wafers together, standing them on edge around outer edge of round serving platter to form a ring. Spread with the remaining pudding mixture. Refrigerate 6 hours or overnight.

Crush remaining 5 wafers; sprinkle over dessert. Make chocolate curls. Top with the chocolate curls. Fill center of ring with strawberries. Store leftover dessert in refrigerator.

Gluten Free Macadamia Pie Crust

Ingredients

6 ounces macadamia nuts
2 eggs
1 1/2 cups soy flour

Directions

Preheat the oven to 350 degrees F (175 degrees C).

Place the macadamia nuts into the container of a food processor, and blend until they reach a peanut butter like consistency. Scrape out into a bowl, and stir in the eggs and soy flour until well blended.

Place the dough between two pieces of waxed paper, and roll out into about a 12 inch circle. Remove the top piece of waxed paper, and invert the dough into a 9 inch pie plate. Press into the bottom and up the sides. Remove any overhanging dough.

Bake for 5 minutes in the preheated oven, or until light golden brown. Use in any recipe calling for a prebaked pie crust.

Double Peanut Butter Cookies I

Ingredients

1 1/2 cups sifted all-purpose flour
1 tablespoon milk
1/2 cup white sugar
1/2 teaspoon baking soda
1/4 cup light corn syrup 1/4
teaspoon salt
1/2 cup shortening
1 cup peanut butter
1 cup semisweet chocolate chips

Directions

Combine flour, sugar, soda and salt. Cut in shortening and peanut butter until mixture resembles coarse meal. Blend in syrup and milk.

Shape in roll 2 inches in diameter; chill. Slice 1/8 to 1/4 inches thick.

Place 1/2 the slices on ungreased cookie sheet; spread each with 1/2 teaspoon peanut butter. Sprinkle chocolate chips on top of the peanut butter. Cover with remaining cookie slices; seal edges with a fork.

Cover with remaining cookie slices; seal edges with a fork. Bake at 350 degrees F (175 degrees C) for 12 minutes, or until browned.

Gramma's Easy Peanut Butter Fudge

Ingredients

1 1/3 cups milk
2 pounds brown sugar
1/4 cup margarine
1 1/2 cups peanut butter
1 teaspoon vanilla extract

Directions

In a medium saucepan over medium heat, combine milk and sugar. Heat to between 234 and 240 degrees F (112 to 116 degrees C), or until a small amount of syrup dropped into cold water forms a soft ball that flattens when removed from the water and placed on a flat surface.

Remove from the heat and stir in margarine, peanut butter and vanilla. Quickly spread into a 9x13 inch dish. Allow to cool almost completely before cutting into squares. Store in an airtight container.

Sugar Free Peanut Butter Balls

Ingredients

1 cup margarine
2 tablespoons granulated artificial sweetener
1 teaspoon vanilla extract
2 tablespoons water
2 cups all-purpose flour
1 egg white
1/2 cup chopped peanuts

Directions

Preheat oven to 350 degrees F (175 degrees C).

Beat margarine and sugar till fluffy. Add vanilla, water, and flour, mixing well. Refrigerate 1 hour.

Form into 1 inch balls, dip into beaten egg white and roll into peanuts. Place on ungreased cookie sheets. Bake 10 to 12 minutes. Store in an airtight container.

Thanksgiving Drumstick Treats™

Ingredients

3 tablespoons butter or margarine
1 (10 ounce) package regular marshmallows
6 cups Kellogg's® Rice Krispies®
Peanut butter
Kellogg's® Cocoa Krispies®

Directions

In large saucepan melt butter over low heat. Add marshmallows and stir until completely melted. Remove from heat.

Add KELLOGG'S RICE KRISPIES cereal. Stir until well coated.

Cool slightly. Using buttered hands shape mixture into twelve small drumsticks.

Spread peanut butter on large end of each drumstick, then dip in KELLOGG'S COCOA KRISPIES cereal. Refrigerate until firm. Best if served the same day.

Slow Cooker Mussaman Curry

Ingredients

2 potatoes, cut into large chunks
1 small onion, coarsely chopped
2 tablespoons butter
1 1/4 pounds beef chuck, cut into 1-inch cubes
3 cloves garlic, minced
1 (14 ounce) can coconut milk
1/4 cup peanut butter
3 tablespoons curry powder
3 tablespoons Thai fish sauce
3 tablespoons brown sugar
2 cups beef broth
1/2 cup unsalted, dry-roasted peanuts

Directions

Place the potatoes and onion in a slow cooker.

Melt the butter in a skillet over medium-high heat. Cook the beef and garlic together in the melted butter until the beef is browned on all sides. Transfer the beef and garlic to the slow cooker while keeping the beef drippings in the skillet.

Return the skillet to the medium-high heat. Stir the coconut milk, peanut butter, and curry powder into the reserved beef drippings; cook and stir until the peanut butter melts. Pour the coconut milk mixture into the slow cooker. Turn the slow cooker on to Low; stir the fish sauce, brown sugar, and beef broth into the slow cooker.

Cook on Low until the beef is fork-tender, 4 to 6 hours. Stir the peanuts into the curry about 30 minutes before serving.

JIF® Festive Fudge

Ingredients

1/3 cup JIF® Reduced Fat Peanut Butter
1 1/2 cups granulated sugar
1 cup marshmallow creme
1/2 cup evaporated milk 1/2 teaspoon salt
1 (6 ounce) package semi-sweet chocolate chips
1 teaspoon vanilla
1/2 cup white chocolate chips 1/2 teaspoon CRISCO® Butter Flavor All-Vegetable Shortening
Colored gumdrops

Directions

Grease 8-inch pan.

Combine sugar, marshmallow creme, milk, JIF® Reduced Fat Peanut Butter and salt in a large saucepan. Stir constantly on low heat until blended and mixture comes to a boil. Boil 5 minutes, stirring constantly. Remove from heat. Add semi-sweet chocolate chips. Stir until well blended. Stir in vanilla. Pour into pan. Cool.

Cut into squares or with cookie cutters.

Melt white chocolate chips with CRISCO® Butter Flavor All-Vegetable Shortening in microwave, stirring at 20-second intervals, until smooth (1-2 minutes). Place mixture in zip top bag. Cut a tiny piece off bottom corner to create a pastry bag. (If chocolate hardens, place in microwave for 7-10 seconds).

Decorate fudge to look like gifts. Uses x's or zigzags to make ribbons and or patterns.

Cut colored gumdrops into slivers. Gather a multi-colored "bouquet" of slivers and press the "stems" into the candies. Place each piece of decorated fudge in a candy cup, place in a gift box.

Sherry Chicken Curry

Ingredients

2 tablespoons vegetable oil
4 skinless, boneless chicken breast halves - cut into chunks
1/2 cup cornstarch
3 cloves garlic, crushed
1 large onion, cut into chunks
salt and pepper to taste
1/2 cup cooking sherry
2 cubes beef bouillon
1/2 cup creamy peanut butter
3 tablespoons curry powder
water to cover
1/2 teaspoon ground ginger
1 cup coconut milk

Directions

Heat oil in a large skillet over medium high heat. Coat chicken with cornstarch and place in skillet with garlic, onion, salt and pepper. Add sherry and beef bouillon and let liquid reduce a little.

Stir in peanut butter and curry powder and add water to cover; add ginger, reduce heat to low and simmer for 30 minutes, then lastly stir in coconut milk and serve hot.

JIF® Peanut Butter Bread

Ingredients

Crisco® Original No-Stick Cooking Spray
2 cups Pillsbury BEST® All Purpose Flour
1/2 cup sugar
2 teaspoons baking powder
1 teaspoon salt
3/4 cup JIF® Creamy Peanut Butter
1 large egg, beaten
1 cup milk

Directions

Heat oven to 350 degrees F. Spray a 9x3x5-inch loaf pan with no-stick cooking spray.

Mix flour, sugar, baking powder and salt in large bowl.

Cut in peanut butter with a fork. Add egg and milk; stir just enough to moisten dry ingredients. Pour into prepared pan.

Bake 60 minutes or until wooden pick inserted near center comes out clean. Cool in pan 10 minutes. Invert and remove loaf to cooling rack.

Chocolate Marshmallow Squares

Ingredients

1 1/2 teaspoons butter
1 (12 ounce) package semisweet chocolate chips
1 (11 ounce) package butterscotch chips
1/2 cup peanut butter
1 (16 ounce) package miniature marshmallows
1 cup unsalted dry roasted peanuts

Directions

Line a 13-in. x 9-in. x 2-in. baking pan with foil and grease the foil with 1-1/2 teaspoons butter; set aside. In a large microwave-safe bowl, microwave the chocolate chips, butterscotch chips and peanut butter at 70% power for 2 minutes; stir. Microwave in 10- to 20-second intervals until melted; stir until smooth. Cool for 1 minute. Stir in marshmallows and peanuts.

Spread into prepared pan. Refrigerate until firm. Using foil, lift candy out of pan. Discard foil; cut into 1-1/2-in. squares.

Peanut Butter Chocolate Sandwich Cookies

Ingredients

1 1/4 cups unbleached all-purpose flour
1/2 teaspoon baking soda
1/2 teaspoon salt
1/2 cup unsalted butter
1/2 cup smooth peanut butter
1 cup white sugar
1 egg
1 tablespoon milk
6 (1 ounce) squares semisweet chocolate
2 teaspoons butter

Directions

In a large bowl mix together the butter until soft. Add the peanut butter and sugar and beat well. Mix in the egg and milk. Sift together the flour, salt, and baking soda. Add to the egg mixture slowly and mix until just blended. Form dough into 2 logs, and wrap in plastic wrap. Freeze for at least 2 hours.

Preheat oven to 375 degrees F (190 degrees C). Grease cookie sheets.

Chop chocolate into small pieces and place in the top of a double boiler over medium heat. Stir frequently until melted. Add butter or margarine and stir until melted. Remove from heat and let cool to room temperature.

Remove one package of the dough from the freezer and unwrap. With a sharp, serrated knife, cut a few slices of the dough 1/4 inch thick and place on cookie sheet about 2 inches apart.

Quickly spoon a teaspoonful of the chocolate on each slice. Cut more slices, and top each with another slice of dough. If dough becomes too soft, rewrap it and return to freezer. Reheat chocolate if it becomes too hard.

Bake 10 to 12 minutes until lightly colored.

Honey Wheat Cookies

Ingredients

1/2 cup butter or margarine, softened
1/2 cup natural peanut butter
1/2 cup honey
1 egg
1 tablespoon vanilla extract
1 cup sifted whole wheat flour
1/2 cup dry milk powder
1/2 cup wheat bran
1 teaspoon baking soda

Directions

Preheat the oven to 350 degrees F (175 degrees C).

In a medium bowl, mix together the butter and peanut butter until smooth. Mix in the honey, egg and vanilla. Combine the whole wheat flour, dry milk powder, wheat bran and baking soda; stir into the peanut butter mixture. Drop by teaspoonfuls onto ungreased baking sheets.

Bake for 8 to 10 minutes in the preheated oven, or until edges begin to brown. Remove from baking sheet to cool on wire racks.

Apple Ladybug Treats

Ingredients

2 red apples
1/4 cup raisins
1 tablespoon peanut butter
8 thin pretzel sticks

Directions

Slice apples in half from top to bottom and scoop out the cores using a knife or melon baller. If you have an apple corer, core them first, then slice. Place each apple half flat side down on a small plate.

Dab peanut butter on to the back of the 'lady bug', then stick raisins onto the dabs for spots. Use this method to make eyes too. Stick one end of each pretzel stick into a raisin, then press the other end into the apples to make antennae.

Fruit and Yogurt Treats

Ingredients

1/3 cup SMUCKER'S®
Strawberry Low Sugar Preserves
1/4 cup JIF® Creamy Peanut
Butter & Honey
1 cup low-fat vanilla yogurt
8 sugar cones
4 cups fresh mixed fruits:
chopped strawberries, bananas,
pineapple, mandarin oranges, kiwi
and blueberries

Directions

Combine preserves, peanut butter and yogurt until blended.

Chop fruit small. Place a tablespoon of yogurt mixture into bottom of cone. Fill cone with fruit until heaping. Top fruit with a dollop of yogurt mixture.

Rayna's Peanut Butter Jammies

Ingredients

8 slices bread
1/2 cup peanut butter
1/4 cup any flavor fruit jam
1 egg, beaten
1/2 cup milk
2 teaspoons white sugar
1 pinch salt
2 tablespoons butter

Directions

Spread four slices of bread with peanut butter and jam. Cover with remaining four slices of bread. Beat together egg, milk, sugar and salt.

In a large skillet or frying pan, melt butter over medium heat.

Dip each sandwich into the egg mixture to coat it well and allow the excess to drip off. Place sandwiches in pan and cook until golden on both sides. Serve warm.

Chocolate Peanut Butter Cup Cookies

Ingredients

1 cup butter, softened
3/4 cup creamy peanut butter
3/4 cup white sugar
3/4 cup packed brown sugar
2 eggs
1 teaspoon vanilla extract
2 1/3 cups all-purpose flour
1/3 cup cocoa powder
1 teaspoon baking soda
1 cup semisweet chocolate chips
1 cup peanut butter chips
10 chocolate covered peanut butter cups, cut into eighths

Directions

Preheat oven to 350 degrees F (175 degrees C).

In a large bowl, cream together the butter, peanut butter, white sugar, and brown sugar until smooth. Beat in the eggs one at a time, then stir in the vanilla. Combine the flour, cocoa, and baking soda; stir into the peanut butter mixture. Mix in the chocolate chips, peanut butter chips, and peanut butter cups. Drop by tablespoonfuls onto ungreased cookie sheets.

Bake for 8 to 10 minutes in the preheated oven. Let cool for 1 or 2 minutes on sheet before removing, or they will fall apart.

Peanut Butter and Banana Smoothie

Ingredients

1 banana
1/8 cup peanut butter
1/2 cup soy milk
2 tablespoons honey

Directions

In a blender, combine banana, peanut butter and soy milk. Blend until smooth. Pour into glasses and drizzle with honey for garnish.

Bun Bars

Ingredients

2 cups semisweet chocolate chips
2 cups butterscotch chips
2 1/2 cups creamy peanut butter
2/3 cup milk
1 cup butter
1 (3.5 ounce) package instant vanilla pudding mix
2 tablespoons confectioners' sugar
3 cups salted peanuts

Directions

Melt butterscotch and chocolate chips and peanut butter until smooth on low to medium heat. Spread half of mixture into the bottom of 9 x 13 inch pan. Chill until hard in freezer.

Melt butter, add instant pudding and milk, boil one minute. Add confectioners' sugar and mix well. It will look funny, but it will mix together.

Put on top of chocolate layer. Chill in the freezer until hard.

Add peanuts to rest of chocolate mixture and spread on top of vanilla layer. Chill in freezer 1 hour until set. Keep in refrigerator until served.

The Whole Jar of Peanut Butter Cookies

Ingredients

1 cup butter, softened
1 cup white sugar
1 cup packed brown sugar 2 egg
1 egg yolk
2 teaspoons vanilla extract
1 (18 ounce) jar peanut butter
2 cups all-purpose flour
1 teaspoon baking soda
1/2 teaspoon salt
1 cup chopped peanuts

Directions

In a large bowl, cream butter, white sugar, and brown sugar until smooth. Add the eggs, yolks, and vanilla; mix until fluffy. Stir in peanut butter. Sift together the flour, baking soda, and salt; stir into the peanut butter mixture. Finally, stir in the peanuts. Refrigerate the dough for at least 2 hours.

Preheat oven to 350 degrees F (175 degrees C). Lightly grease a cookie sheet.

Roll dough into walnut sized balls. Place on the prepared cookie sheet and flatten slightly with a fork. Bake for 12 to 15 minutes in the preheated oven. Cookies should look dry on top. Allow to cool for a few minutes on the cookie sheet before removing to cool completely on a rack. These cookies taste great when slightly undercooked.

Odd Bagel Sandwiches

Ingredients

2 tablespoons peanut butter
1 bagel, split and toasted
4 slices sliced pepperoni

Directions

Spread the peanut butter on the bagel while still warm. Arrange the pepperoni on the peanut butter and sandwich between the 2 bagel halves.

Flourless Peanut Butter Cookies

Ingredients

4 egg whites
2 cups peanut butter
1 2/3 cups sugar

Directions

In a mixing bowl, beat egg whites until stiff peaks form. In another bowl, combine peanut butter and sugar; fold in egg whites. Drop by heaping teaspoonfuls 2 in. apart onto lightly greased baking sheets. Flatten slightly with a fork. Bake at 325 degrees F for 15-20 minutes or until set. Remove to wire racks to cool.

Peanut Butter Ice Cream Topping

Ingredients

1 cup white sugar
1/2 cup water
1/2 cup peanut butter

Directions

Mix together the white sugar and water in a small saucepan over high heat and bring to a boil; boil for one minute. Remove from heat and stir in the peanut butter until melted well blended. Pour the warm sauce over ice cream to serve.

My Favorite Sesame Noodles

Ingredients

1/2 (8 ounce) package spaghetti
2 tablespoons peanut butter
1 tablespoon honey
2 tablespoons tamari
1 teaspoon Thai chili sauce
1 teaspoon sesame oil
1 teaspoon ground ginger
1 clove garlic, minced
1 green onion, chopped
2 teaspoons sesame seeds

Directions

Fill a large pot with lightly salted water and bring to a rolling boil over high heat. Once the water is boiling, stir in the spaghetti, and return to a boil. Cook the pasta uncovered, stirring occasionally, until the pasta has cooked through, but is still firm to the bite, about 12 minutes. Drain well in a colander set in the sink.

Melt the peanut butter in a large microwave-safe glass or ceramic bowl, 15 to 20 seconds (depending on your microwave). Whisk the honey, tamari, and chili sauce into the peanut butter, then stir in the sesame oil and ginger. Mix in the garlic and green onions and toss with the spaghetti. Top with the sesame seeds.

Peanut Butter Pie IV

Ingredients

1 (8 ounce) package cream cheese
1 (14 ounce) can sweetened condensed milk
3/4 cup peanut butter
3 tablespoons lemon juice
1 teaspoon vanilla extract
1 cup frozen whipped topping, thawed
1 (9 inch) prepared graham cracker crust
2 tablespoons chocolate syrup

Directions

Beat cream cheese until fluffy. Beat in milk and peanut butter until smooth. Stir in lemon juice and vanilla. Fold in whipped topping.

Pour filling into crust. Drizzle syrup over the filling, and swirl. Chill.

Shrimp and Peanut Butter Noodles

Ingredients

1/4 cup peanut butter
2 tablespoons light soy sauce
2 tablespoons Chinese black vinegar
2 tablespoons white sugar
1 tablespoon sesame oil
10 ounces dried Japanese udon noodles
20 uncooked large shrimp - peeled, deveined, tails left intact
1 cup broccoli florets
1/4 cup chopped roasted peanuts (optional)

Directions

In a small bowl, mix together the peanut butter, soy sauce, black vinegar, sugar, and sesame oil. Set aside.

Bring a large pot of water to a boil. Stir in the udon noodles and cook for 5 minutes. Add the frozen shrimp to the pot of boiling noodles and cook for about 3 minutes, until the shrimp are pink and opaque. Turn the stove off, but do not remove pot from the heat. Stir in the broccoli, cover, and let sit for 2-3 minutes.

Drain the noodles, broccoli, and shrimp. In a large serving bowl, toss together the noodles, broccoli, shrimp, and the peanut butter sauce. Garnish with chopped peanuts.

Franks in Peanut Butter and Chutney

Ingredients

3/4 cup creamy peanut butter
1/2 cup chutney
1 1/2 cups chicken stock
3 tablespoons light corn syrup
3 tablespoons soy sauce
2 cloves crushed garlic
2 pounds hot dogs

Directions

Cut each frank into five bite-sized pieces, unless you're using cocktail wieners.

In a large saucepan, combine peanut butter, chutney, chicken stock, corn syrup, Heat and stir constantly until very smooth. Add franks and continue stirring carefully until franks are covered with sauce. Reduce heat and continue to heat slowly until franks are hot. Insert toothpicks into frankfurters and serve.

Honey-Peanut Butter Cookies

Ingredients

1/2 cup shortening
1 cup creamy peanut butter
1 cup honey
2 eggs, lightly beaten
3 cups all-purpose flour
1 cup sugar
1 1/2 teaspoons baking soda
1 teaspoon baking powder
1/2 teaspoon salt

Directions

In a mixing bowl, mix shortening, peanut butter and honey. Add eggs; mix well. Combine flour, sugar, baking soda, baking powder and salt; add to peanut butter mixture and mix well.

Roll into 1- to 1-1/2-in. balls and place on ungreased baking sheets. Flatten with a fork dipped in flour. Bake at 350 degrees F for 8-10 minutes.

Coconut Curry Black Bean Burgers - Thai Style!

Ingredients

1 (15 ounce) can black beans, rinsed and drained
1 tablespoon finely chopped red onion
1 clove garlic, minced
1/2 teaspoon salt
1 teaspoon Thai chile sauce
1 teaspoon yellow curry paste
2 tablespoons coconut milk
1 teaspoon brown sugar
1 pinch cayenne pepper
1 egg
1 cup Italian bread crumbs
1 (1 pound) package crumbled tofu
1 (12 ounce) package vegetarian burger crumbles

1 cup chunky peanut butter
1 teaspoon Thai chile sauce
1 teaspoon brown sugar
1/2 teaspoon salt
1/2 teaspoon ground turmeric
1 dash soy sauce (optional)
1 tablespoon canola oil

6 whole wheat hamburger buns
1/2 cup shredded carrots
1/2 cup shredded cucumber
1 tablespoon chopped green onion
2 tablespoons fresh mint leaves
2 tablespoons fresh cilantro leaves

Directions

Blend the black beans, red onion, garlic, 1/2 teaspoon salt, 1 teaspoon chile sauce, curry paste, coconut milk, 1 teaspoon brown sugar, cayenne pepper, and egg in a food processor until smooth. Scrape the mixture into a large bowl. Fold the bread crumbs and burger crumbles into the mixture. Form the mixture into 6 patties and place on waxed paper. Put in freezer for up to 30 minutes for patties to set.

Prepare a grill pan or skillet with cooking spray and place over medium heat. Cook the patties until browned, 4 to 5 minutes per side.

Meanwhile, combine the peanut butter, 1 teaspoon chile sauce, 1 teaspoon brown sugar, 1/2 teaspoon salt, turmeric, soy sauce, and canola oil in a saucepan over medium-low heat. Cook and stir until the peanut butter is melted. Reduce heat to low and simmer until hot, 3 to 5 minutes.

Arrange patties on bottoms of hamburger buns. Drizzle sauce over each patty; top with carrot, cucumber, green onion, mint, and cilantro. Top with remaining bun halves and serve immediately.

Peanut Butter Cookies

Ingredients

3 tablespoons butter
2 tablespoons reduced fat peanut butter
1/2 cup packed brown sugar
1/4 cup sugar
1 egg white
1 teaspoon vanilla extract
1 cup all-purpose flour 1/4 teaspoon baking soda 1/8 teaspoon salt

Directions

In a large mixing bowl, cream the butter, peanut butter and sugars. Add egg white; beat until blended. Beat in vanilla. Combine flour, baking soda and salt; gradually add to the creamed mixture. Shape into an 8-in. roll; wrap in plastic wrap. Freeze for 2 hours or until firm.

Unwrap and cut into slices, about 1/4 in. thick. Place 2 in. apart on baking sheets coated with nonstick cooking spray. flatten with a fork. Bake at 350 degrees F for 6-8 minutes for chewy cookies or 8 -10 minutes for crisp cookies. Cool for 1-2 minutes before removing to wire racks; cool completely.

PB&J Bars

Ingredients

1 (18 ounce) package refrigerated sugar cookie dough, divided
2/3 cup strawberry jam
3/4 cup granola without raisins
3/4 cup peanut butter chips

Directions

Line a 9-in. square baking pan with foil and greased the foil. Press two-thirds of the cookie dough into prepared pan. Spread jam over dough to within 1/4 in. of edges. In a mixing bowl, beat the granola, peanut butter chips and remaining dough until blended. Crumble over jam.

Bake at 375 degrees F for 25-30 minutes or until golden brown. Cool on a wire rack. Using foil, lift out of pan. Cut into bars and remove from foil.

S'more Sandwiches

Ingredients

2 slices bread
2 tablespoons peanut butter
2 teaspoons butter
2 tablespoons milk chocolate chips
1/4 cup miniature marshmallows

Directions

Spread butter onto one side of each slice of bread. Place bread butter sides down in the pie iron. Spread half of the peanut butter onto the exposed side of each piece of bread. Stick the marshmallows to one side and the chocolate chips to the other. Close the pie maker.

Roast over a campfire for about 3 minutes on each side, until the bread is toasted. It should be nice and golden like a grilled cheese with chips melted and marshmallows gooey.

Indian Peanut Stew

Ingredients

2 cups uncooked brown rice
6 cups water
1 tablespoon olive oil
1 large white onion, chopped
4 cloves garlic, minced
3 tablespoons grated fresh ginger root
1 (28 ounce) can diced tomatoes with juice
1/8 teaspoon cayenne pepper
1 cup chunky natural peanut butter

Directions

Place rice and water in a large saucepan and bring to a boil. Cover, and reduce heat to low. Simmer until rice is tender and water has absorbed, about 30 minutes.

Heat olive oil in a large saucepan over medium-low heat. Add onion, and cook until soft and golden, stirring frequently. Add garlic and ginger, and cook until fragrant, about 5 minutes. Stir in tomatoes, and season with cayenne pepper. Increase heat to medium, and bring to a gentle simmer. Stir in peanut butter and heat through. The mixture will thicken. Serve over rice.

Ingredients

1 1/2 cups butter, softened
1 1/4 cups packed brown sugar
1 1/4 cups white sugar
1 egg
1 teaspoon vanilla extract
4 cups all-purpose flour
2 teaspoons baking soda
1/2 teaspoon salt
1 cup semisweet chocolate chips
1 cup peanut butter chips

Directions

Preheat oven to 350 degrees F (175 degrees C).

In a large bowl, cream together the butter, brown sugar and white sugar until light and fluffy. Beat in the egg, then stir in the vanilla. Combine the flour, baking soda and salt; gradually stir into the creamed mixture. Finally, stir in the chocolate and peanut butter chips. Drop by rounded spoonfuls onto the unprepared cookie sheet.

Bake for 8 to 10 minutes in the preheated oven. Allow cookies to cool on baking sheet for 5 minutes before removing to a wire rack to cool completely.

Peanut Butter Loaf

Ingredients

1 3/4 cups all-purpose flour
1 teaspoon baking soda
1/2 teaspoon salt
1 cup brown sugar
1/3 cup peanut butter
1 egg, beaten
1/2 teaspoon vanilla extract
1 cup buttermilk

Directions

Preheat oven to 350 degrees F (175 degrees C). Lightly grease an 8x4 inch baking pan.

Sift together flour, soda and salt. In a large bowl, cream sugar and peanut butter together. Beat in egg and vanilla until smooth. Stir in flour and milk alternately, beating until smooth after each addition. Spoon batter into prepared pan.

Bake in preheated oven for 1 hour, until well browned. Remove from the pan to cool. Store in a covered container.

Rocky Road

Ingredients

2 cups semisweet chocolate chips
1 cup peanut butter
4 cups miniature marshmallows

Directions

Grease a 9 x 9 inch pan.

Heat chocolate chips and peanut butter over low heat in a medium saucepan until chips are completely melted. Remove from heat. Stir in marshmallows.

Pour into prepared pan. Cool. Can be put into refrigerator to cool. Cut and Enjoy!

Peanut Butter and Jelly Roll-Ups

Ingredients

1 (3 ounce) package low fat cream cheese, softened
1/2 cup SMUCKER'S Strawberry Low Sugar Preserves, (or any of your favorite SMUCKER'S Low Sugar or Sugar Free Preserves
4 whole wheat or flour tortillas
2/3 cup JIF® Creamy Peanut Butter

Directions

Combine softened cream cheese and preserves in a small bowl until well blended.

Spread tortillas with peanut butter to within 1/2 inch of edges of tortillas.

Top peanut butter with cream cheese mixture, to within 1/2 inch of edges. Carefully roll up the tortillas.

Wrap each rolled tortilla securely in plastic wrap. Refrigerate for several hours or overnight. To serve, remove from refrigerator and unwrap. Slice each tortilla into 4-8 angled slices.

CPSIA information can be obtained
at www.ICGtesting.com
Printed in the USA
BVHW061946180521
607636BV00012B/1559